THE TIMES OF INDIA

Jaldi fit KIDS

with namita jain

10 food & fitness mantras

for children from 4 to 14

A must-read for every parent

Times Group Books

Author
Namita Jain

Consultant
Geeta Gopalakrishnan

Copy Editor
Madhuri Iyer

Cover and Book Design
Kermin Sean Colaço

Photography
Himanshu Seth

Stylist for Namita
Bhairavi Rajesh Sanghi

DTP
Nilima Mangesh Rawool

Exercise Demonstration
Namita Jain

First Edition 2010

Caution
Always consult your physician before starting any fitness and / or nutrition program.

Marketed & Distributed by

Times Group Books
(A division of Bennett, Coleman and Company Limited)
Times Annexe, 9-10, Bahadur Shah Zafar Marg, New Delhi-110002

Printed at: Tan Prints (India) Pvt. Ltd.

ISBN: 978-81-89906-93-1

Price: ₹295

Foreword

For around 50 years, I have had the privilege of looking after thousands of children. When I was the Medical Director of Jaslok Hospital and Research Centre, Mumbai, I noticed a marked increase in the number of children and young adults becoming obese and developing diabetes, hypertension and early heart attacks. There is ample evidence to show that the increasing incidence of such illnesses is often due to unhealthy food habits and lack of exercise.

Last year, Yogini Mishra, coordinator for the Mumbai based Association for Consumers Action on Safety and Health attended a workshop in Malaysia, the "Kids Lunch Box Challenge." Most of the children who took part in the challenge picked fast food and carbonated drinks instead of nutritious food and water. This indicated that the children were being brainwashed into buying aggressively advertised brands. The same challenge was subsequently held in Mumbai. Findings revealed that 60 percent of school children in Mumbai city opted for junk food.

Healthy foods offer a balanced range of essential nutrients, while unhealthy foods lack these vital ingredients. Packaged foods may even contain chemical additives that could be harmful. A familiar example of an unhealthy fast food meal is a burger, chips and a cold drink, or fried snacks like samosas and kachoris. Refined flour (maida) preparations such as biscuits, cakes, or white bread also lack important nutrients. Moreover, these foods are devoid of fibre and can cause constipation.

I am happy that we have in our midst Namita Jain – a wellness expert. She has realised the dangers of the unhealthy lifestyles invading our homes and sat down to write 'Jaldi Fit Kids' 10 Food & Fitness Mantras - an excellent book to protect our future citizens from the above-mentioned 'silent killers.'

The 10 Food & Fitness Mantras for kids are written with a keen insight into the difficulties that parents face! The book serves as a guide to balance tasty food with the nutritional needs of children.

The four S's of fitness - stamina, strength, suppleness and stability, should be shared with young children. These could possibly inspire children to give exercise its due importance and to incorporate sports into their daily lives.

Every page of this book deserves careful reading. However, to save time, you may like to check the index and concentrate on the crucial segments - kid-friendly kitchens, the food pyramid, energy providers, fibre-rich foods and innovative recipes. If your child is on a tight daily schedule, focus on the 15-minute home strength routine and the 5-minute home activity.

I firmly believe that 'Jaldi Fit Kids' is not only a must-read for every parent in India and abroad but also for family physicians, pediatricians and dieticians who can then recommend it to parents of children under their care. This book will make a valuable supplement to their supervision.

Dr. R.K. Anand
MD (Ped.), FRCP (Edin.), DCH (Lond.), FIAP

Introduction

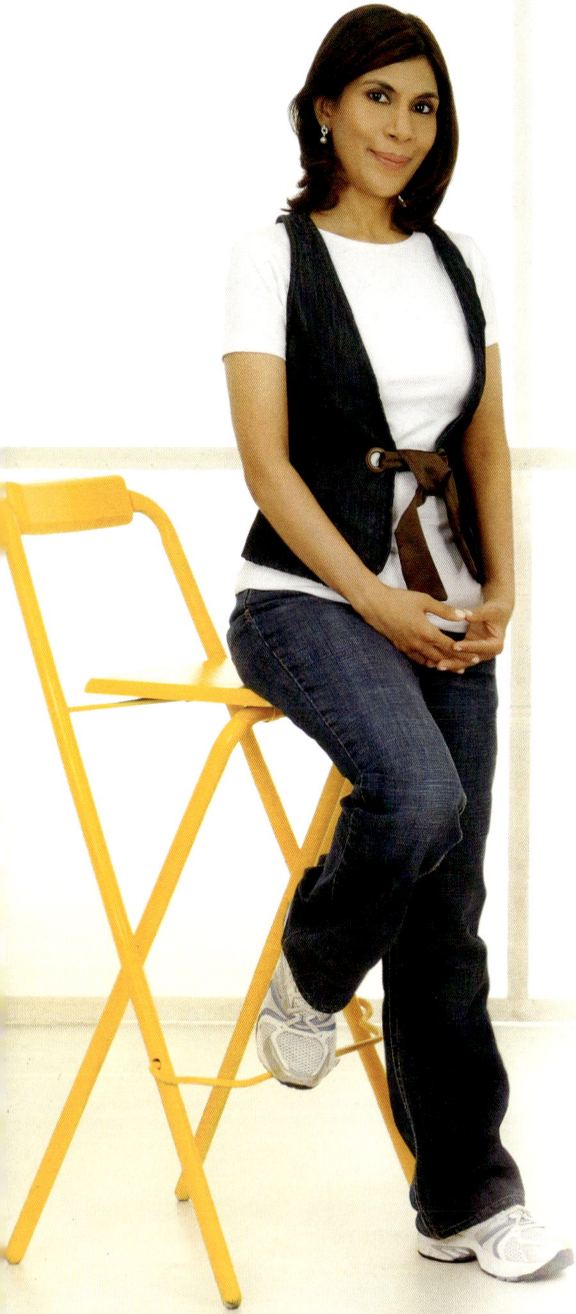

Dear Care Givers, Homework Helpers, Children's Leftovers Finishers, Messy Room Cleaners, Etiquette Minders, Games & Party Organizers, Troubleshooters, 24x7 Disaster Managers, also known as Parents, welcome.

I invite you to open a new chapter in managing your children's health and well being. My 10 Food & Fitness Mantras promise to make your job as a parent simpler and more hassle-free. The idea is to equip you to deal with day to day issues, related to food and fitness.

My 10 Food & Fitness Mantras offer step-by-step guidance to help you instill healthy habits in your kids. This book is especially important now, coming at a time when your children are under fire, bombarded with the impact of 21st century living.

The world over, statistics indicate that children are succumbing to the fast food culture and sedentary lifestyles. Unfortunately, it's happening at the cost of their health. Obesity. Juvenile diabetes. Attention deficit disorder, also known as ADD. Malnutrition. These are just some of the maladies that ail modern children.

While I do not want to sound alarmist, the current trend is cause for deep concern. As a wellness professional, I have seen a steady deterioration in children's health. A couple of decades ago, kids with health problems were anecdotal cases. But in the last 5 years or so, a large segment of children are being clinically defined as "dangerously unfit".

This is because our modern environment, our artificial lifestyle, does not let kids be kids.

In the old days life was simple. Food was made at home and served fresh, and everyone ate together at the family dining table. Today, kids eat out at fast food joints. This means, even when they do eat, they are malnourished, because of nutritional deficiencies.

In times gone by, kids got their exercise by playing hide and seek around the apartment block and walking to school. Now, they step in and out of cars. Or sit in front of the television all evening.

Kids today seem to live on another planet. And parents appear to be fighting a losing battle as children divide their attention between junk food and video games.

But it is never too late to win back lost ground. The 10 Food & Fitness Mantras give your kids a fighting chance!

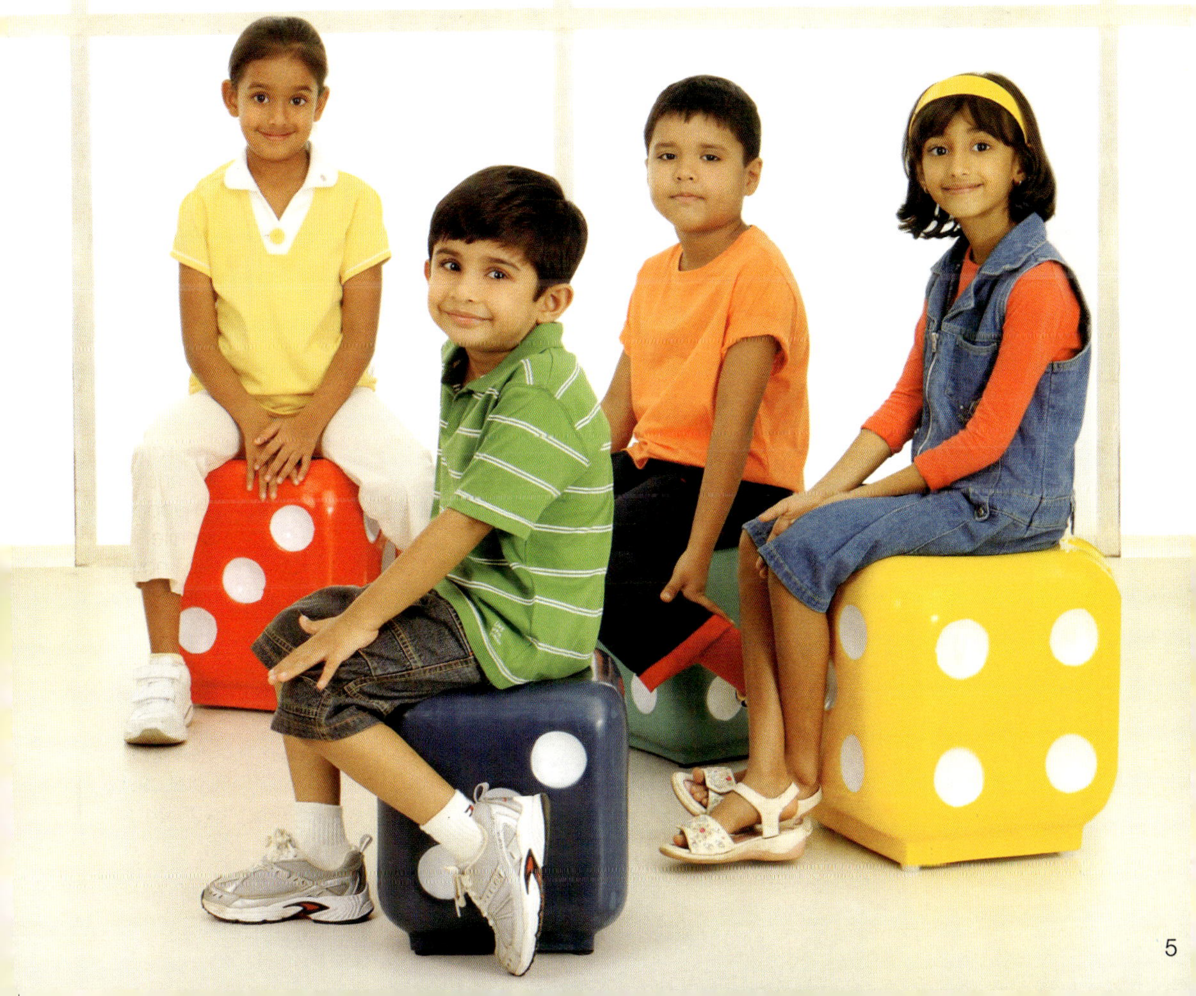

Inculcate good eating habits as your counter-attack against the fast food onslaught. Include a regular exercise regimen to combat obesity.

This two-pronged strategy is detailed in the 10 Food & Fitness Mantras. The first 5 Mantras cover food, and the second half, from Mantras 6 to 10, get into various aspects of fitness.

I am extremely honoured to have the Foreword written by Dr. R. K. Anand. He has endorsed the book as a valuable tool for bringing up a healthy child. Dr. Anand is an eminent child specialist, a Fellow of the Indian Academy of Paediatrics and Fellow of the Royal College of Physicians, Edinburgh. Author of Dr. Anand's Guide to Childcare, he is an authority on the subject.

Namita Jain

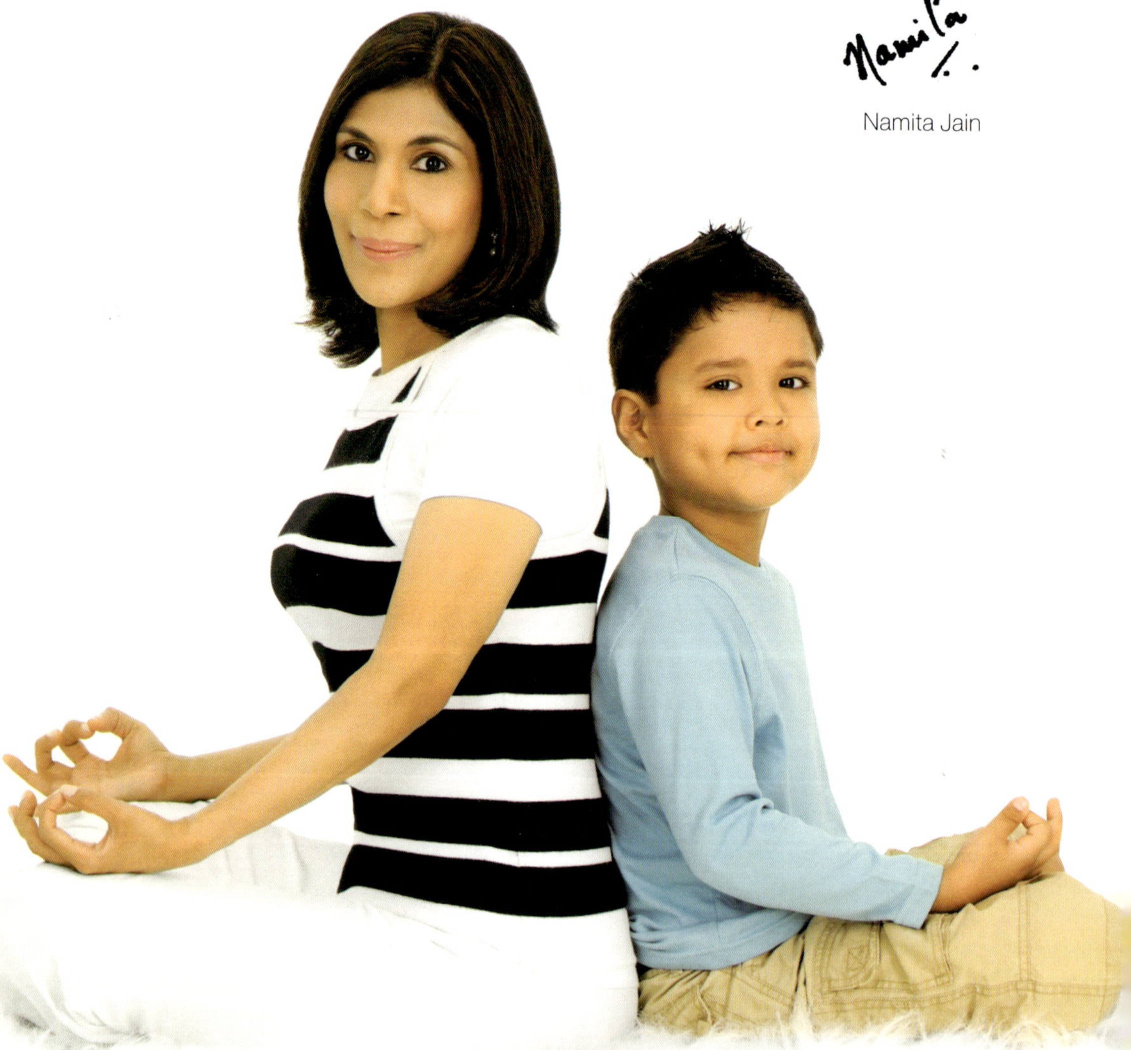

are you ready?

I want to equip you, as a parent, with all the ammunition you need to **fight the fast-food onslaught** and guard your children against obesity and illness.

Use the **10 Food & Fitness Mantras** as your weapons to take up the battle and keep your kids fighting fit!

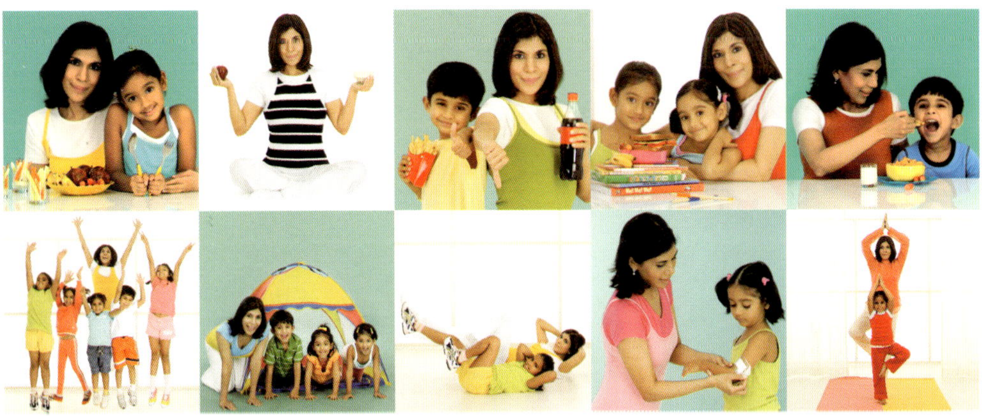

Contents

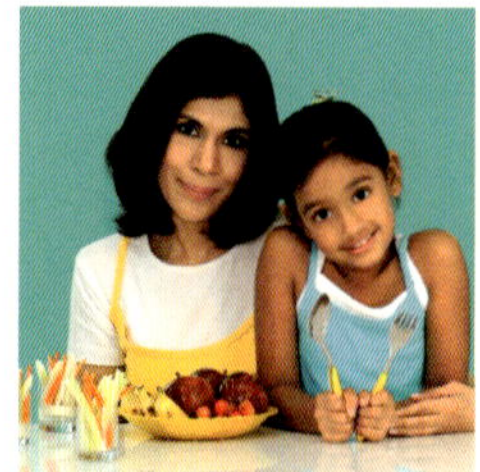

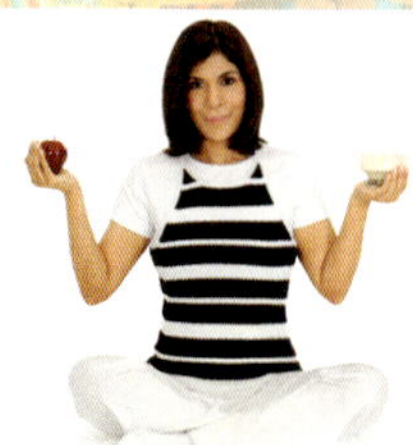

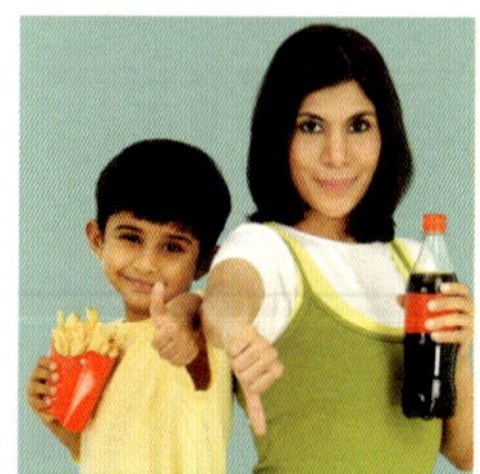

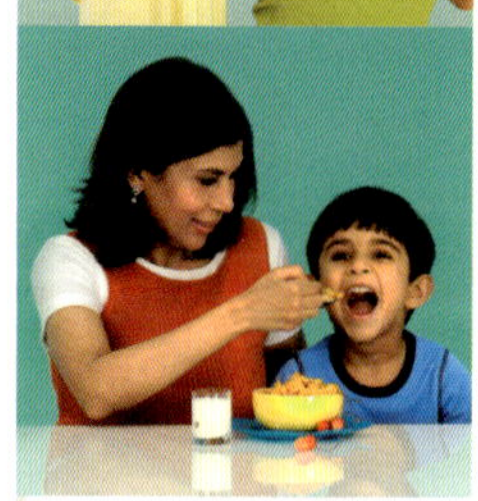

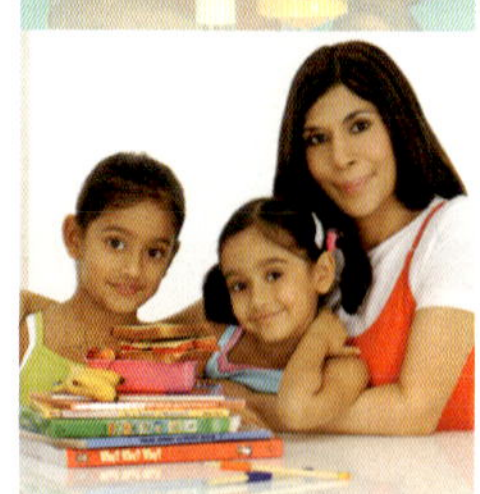

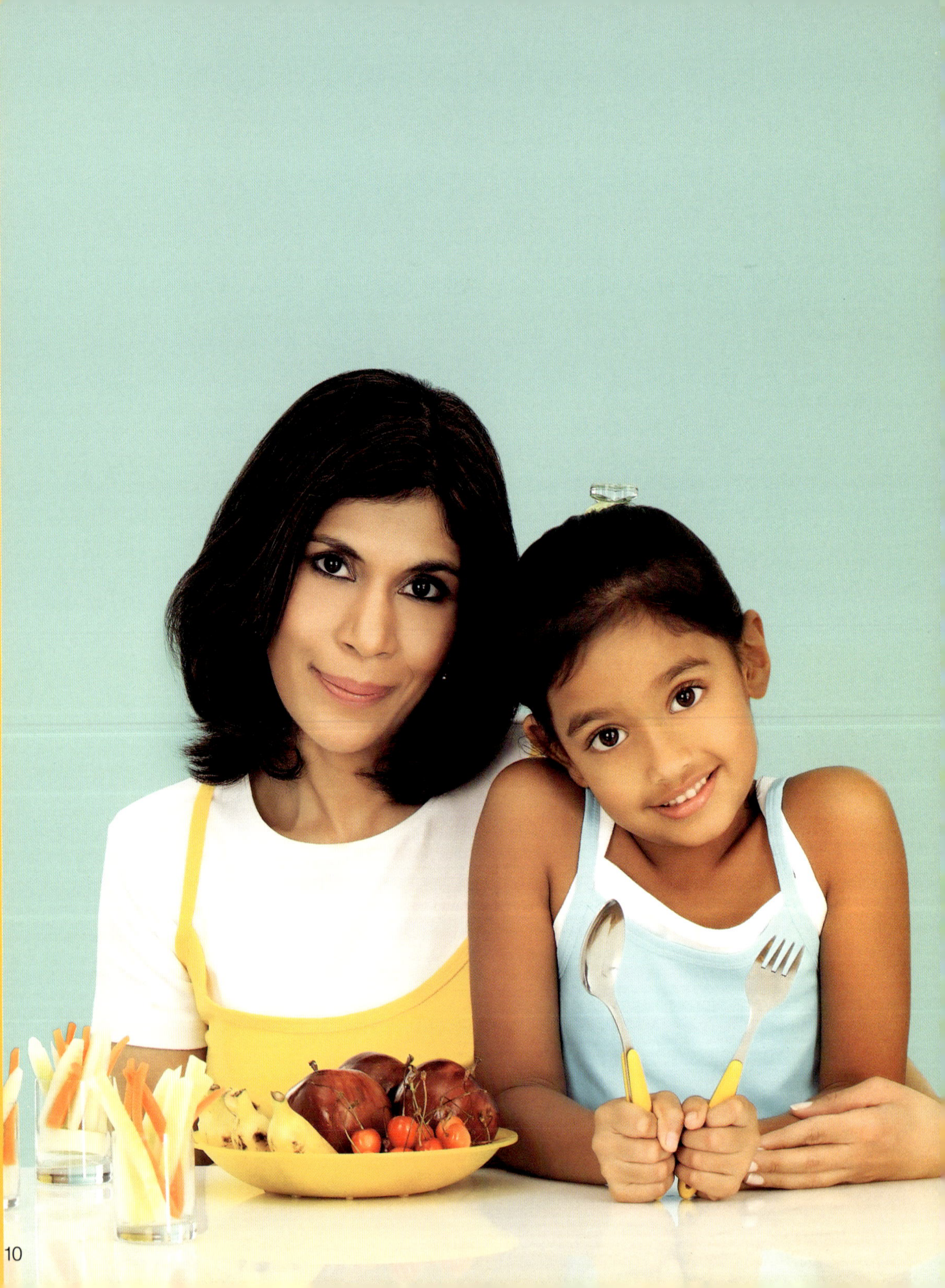

Mantra 1

Good eating habits must develop from an early age. Just as **you teach** your child to walk, to read, or to be **well-behaved,** you can teach your child to eat right.

GROWING UP TO GOOD EATING HABITS

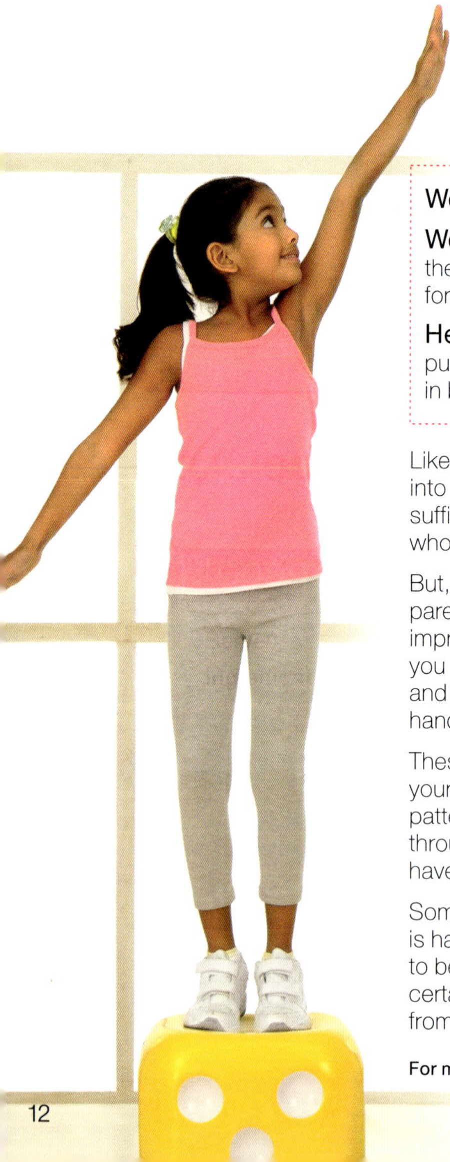

Good eating habits must develop from an early age. Just as you teach your child to walk, to read, or to be well-behaved, you can teach your child to eat right. Good eating habits, once formed, are set for life. Sensible eating, along with a regular, sustained fitness routine, contributes to the overall growth and well being of your child. It is easy to see why mantra 1 is crucial for a happy, healthy childhood.

Growth is a very important indicator of your child's health. Children grow rapidly between 4 to 14 years of age. During this period, their weight almost doubles.

Weights & Measures

Weight On an average, a child gains 2 to 3 kilos per year, until the approach of puberty. The average puberty age is 11 years for girls and around 13 years for boys.

Height A child gains 6 to 8 cm per year from the age of two until puberty. The growth spurt peaks at 12 years in girls and 14 years in boys, then slows to a stop at around 18 years of age.

Like most parents, you want to see your child blossom. To grow into an active healthy toddler. To develop into a smart and self-sufficient student. And finally, to become a bright, confident adult who does you proud.

But, like most parents, you might be at a loss how to go about it. A parent often asks, "Is my child growing properly?" "How can I improve my child's eating habits?" By helping your child to eat well, you are ensuring your child's steady development, both physical and mental, through the growing years. It is a big task you have on hand and sometimes the responsibility can be overwhelming.

These challenges can be overcome if you put a little thought into your child's nutritional needs. While every family has different eating patterns, there is a basic requirement for balanced, healthy meals throughout the day. Even snacks cannot be "empty" - but must have some nutritional value to contribute to healthy growth.

Some kids are poor eaters while others end up eating too much. It is hard for parents to gauge what is "normal". As a parent, you need to be flexible in some situations, but by and large, you can follow certain guidelines to ensure your child picks up good eating habits from an early age.

For more information on good eating habits log on to www.liveactive.com

Answer 'Yes' or 'No' to the statements below to understand your child's eating pattern

- Has regular eating habits Yes☐ No ☐
- Eats when hungry, not out of boredom Yes☐ No ☐
- Is not in the habit of indulging in fried packaged savories every day Yes☐ No ☐
- Eats breakfast every day Yes☐ No ☐
- Eats fruits every day Yes☐ No ☐
- Eats vegetables every day Yes☐ No ☐
- Eats a variety of foods - dairy, wholegrain, vegetables and fruits Yes☐ No ☐
- Does not complain when something new is introduced Yes☐ No ☐
- Drinks adequate quantities of water through the day Yes☐ No ☐
- Enjoys eating wholesome food Yes☐ No ☐

If you have answered 'yes' to most of the statements, you deserve a medal. Right now! Your child is certainly going, or growing, in the right direction. While this is reason to cheer, please keep in mind that children can change their eating habits overnight, or have lean phases, when, for no apparent reason, they cut down on their food.

For the few 'no's' you might have notched up, don't despair. Tact goes a long way in rectifying the areas that need improvement. Go one step at a time. Introduce changes the smart way.

Needs and preferences change with age. From toddler to young adult, your child could take you through a series of perplexing stages that are hard enough to understand, let alone keep pace with. Relax. Go with the flow. Believe me, over time, your sense of humour will stand you in good stead.

Planning Meals

Plan, prepare and pursue good eating habits and you have laid the building blocks for a healthy child. You don't need a degree in nutrition science or in pediatrics to figure out how to go about it! To capture your child's interest and make meal-times something to look forward to, include as much variety, colour and fun as possible. Yes, I said fun. Because, after all, eating is all about enjoyment.

Routine Works Best

Children thrive on routine. Encourage regular eating habits at scheduled times through the day, for snacks and for regular meals. Children eat best when small servings are offered five to six times a day. Contrary to what you might think, your child will actually enjoy wholesome snacks such as fresh fruits, milk, wholegrain crackers, dry cereal - popcorn, kurmura, khakra, idlis, poha, upma and peanut butter sandwiches.

Sometimes, depending on your child's hunger levels, a meal may become a snack, and a snack may become a meal. As long as the food is nutritious, it really does not matter. What is important is, through the course of the day, your child gets adequate nutrition within a 24-hour cycle.

Your child's eating experience is about smell, touch, visual appeal.

How often has your child rejected food because "it smells funny"? Or refused a sandwich because it was "cut the wrong way"? When children accept food, it is not taste alone that helps them decide. Senses like smell and touch play a big role.

Children tend to stay away from strong odours, such as garlic, or avoid food served at extreme temperatures. Children also prefer to identify exactly what they are eating. For example, casseroles, or curries, which mix up lots of different ingredients, are harder for kids to eat, as they do not know what they are eating.

If, by chance, you happen to serve up broken biscuits or hot milk with bits of malai floating in it, be prepared to have it rejected outright!

Age in years	Attitude to food	What you can do
4-7	Food is described by colour, shape and quantity. Foods tend to be categorized into "I like" and "I don't like".	Make mealtimes enjoyable. Try to understand their preferences, work around them and be patient.
7-11	Mealtimes take on a social significance. The expanding environment plays a role in food selection and so does peer influence.	Limit indulgences to occasions or weekends. Be a role model. At this age they are open to learning, so continue educating them on nutritious food and its positive effect on growth and health.
11 and above	Conflict may arise when making food choices. What is good for them versus going out for fast food can be a constant tussle.	Be understanding. Voice your views, yet allow them to make choices. Be neither restrictive nor over-indulgent.

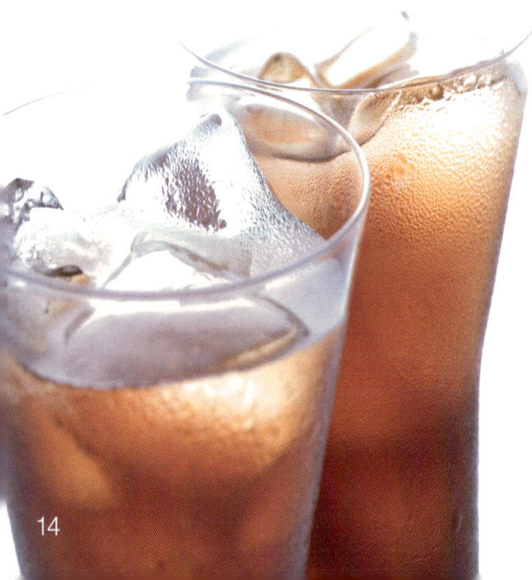

What Parents Say...

One day Maya's son came to her and said that instead of water, he wanted his school water bottle filled with a cola. When Maya asked why, he said his friends were doing so. Instead of raising her voice, Maya patiently explained the benefits of water in the water bottle he was carrying and why a cola was detrimental to his health. Her son realized that just because his friends did it, was no reason for him to do likewise – and that it didn't make them "cool".

As an incentive, his Mom promised him a cola drink on weekends and it was a win win solution for both!

For more information on the benefits of water, refer to my website, www.liveactive.com

FIT Tip

Say yes to sweets, ice cream, chocolates. Indulge, but in moderation. Perhaps you can set a special day like Sunday for once-a-week treats, or offer special goodies on special occasions only.

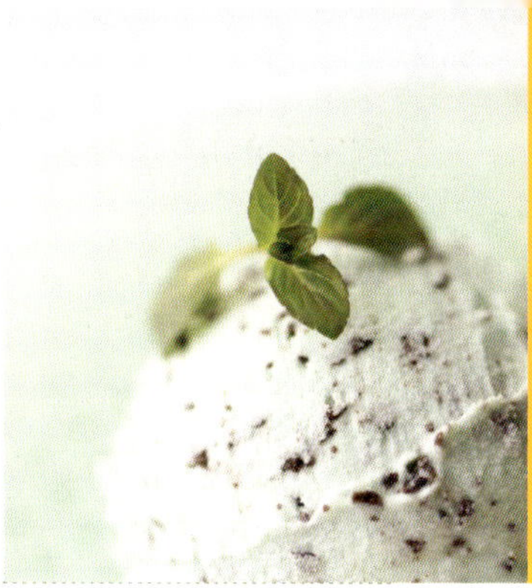

Q: My son takes too long to chew. Should I coax him to eat fast?

A: Allow him to take time over his meal. Chewing is the first stage of digestion. Teeth are designed to grind food into a liquid mush. Get your child into the habit of chewing each mouthful, ideally 20 times for every bite.

Q: I have two children and they always leave unfinished food on their plate. Isn't it important for them to learn not to waste food?

A: Teaching them to clean the plate will not do much for their health. Instead, teach your children to take smaller quantities on their plates. This way, they are able to finish their first helping and can have seconds if they are still hungry.

As a parent, you may feel one small helping is too little. But let me assure you children instinctively know how much to consume. Encourage them to listen to their hunger signals and eat only when they are hungry.

If you insist on your child getting up from the dining table only after finishing everything on the plate, you are disrupting the child's all-important body signals that indicate he or she has had enough. In fact, the more you force a child, the more resistance you are likely to face during meal-times. Instead, just try to make meals pleasant and peaceful, and your children will thank you for it!

FIT Facts

Force feeding never works. Inspiration to eat, as opposed to imposition, does the trick.

Children have individual appetites governed by the appetite centre (appestat) in their brain.

Children need physical activity and time in fresh air to stimulate a good appetite.

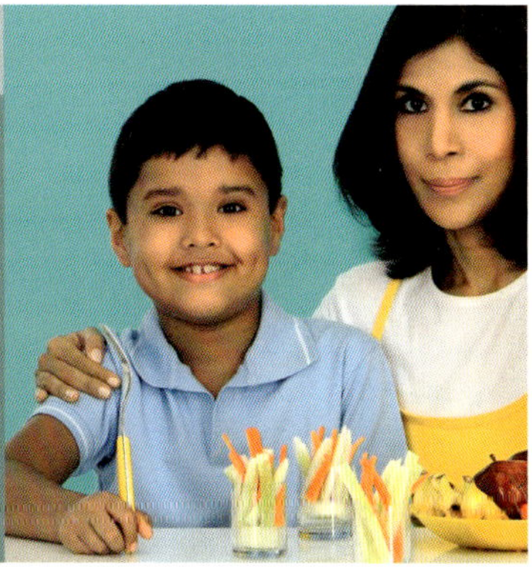

serve up some variety, colour and fun!

VARIETY

When you give your child variety from all the food groups - cereals, dairy products, meat, fruits, vegetables and fats - you are ensuring well-rounded nutrition for your kid. This is the basic template for good health. Once regular, balanced eating patterns are set in childhood, children tend to carry over these habits into adulthood as well.

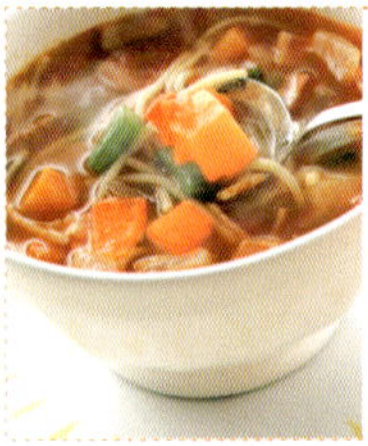

What Parents Say...

You could never dangle a carrot before Saurabh, he literally saw red! It worried his Mum. She served it in a soup and he liked it. Say carrots, and now Saurabh says, "In a soup? Yes!"

- Try a vegetable that you normally do not cook, and encourage your child to try it.
- If your child dislikes a vegetable, don't force it down. Find innovative ways to serve it up. For instance, if cabbage is a no-no, turn a cabbage leaf into a "bowl" with mixed veggies inside it and your child will see it with new eyes!
- If your child is sleepy, do not force food.
- When your child does try something new, make sure you praise the effort.

FACT-O-Meter

It could take as many as 10 attempts before a child accepts new food. Try to keep offering, without forcing your child to consume it, and you may get lucky.

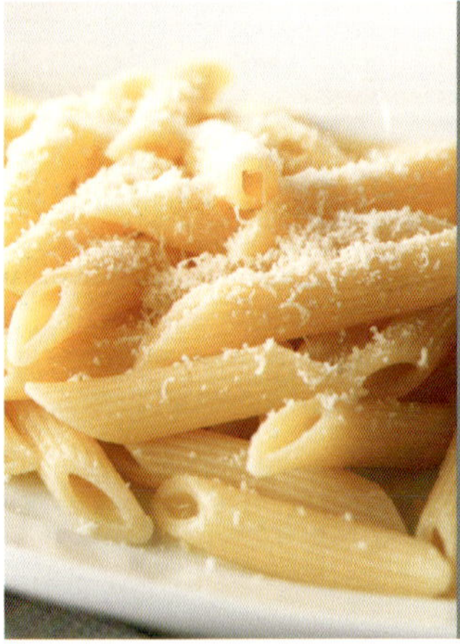

Did you know?

Children need to be exposed to new foods several times before they are willing to try them. Whenever you experiment with something new, you will see the look of anticipation, and maybe some apprehension, on your child's face.

If your child seems reluctant, explain what is special about the dish, where it comes from. For example, compare a pasta dish from Italy with noodles from China – just asking what looks similar about these dishes can start off a great dining table conversation! Make the food look really appetizing as well. Serve it in a colourful dish, garnish it with multi-coloured ingredients like coriander leaves or julienne–cut carrots.

is your child is a fussy eater?

Let's face it, most kids are fussy at one time or another. Luckily, picky eating habits, like many of the quirks of childhood, don't last long. Keep your perspective. Offer your child a wide variety of foods. Encourage, but don't force your child to try them. Just because your son has refused porridge today, it doesn't mean he won't like it next week or next month. The next time you serve porridge, make it different by adding raisins or a fruit.

Often, fussiness is just a phase. If you are too pushy your child may get averse to trying new foods. Sometimes what seems likes fussiness is actually a preference, so try to be sensitive to your child's likes and dislikes. Just like you, they too have their food preferences. As you well know, feeding a child involves a lot of understanding, patience and time.

Let me add here, one more crucial input is creativity! You will be surprised to find that, just as you are ready to give up, a creative, out-of-the-box solution works wonders.

Children who have a long record of fussy eating are usually made that way by over-indulgent parents. If you give in to your child's whims, offering ready alternatives whenever your child makes a fuss, you will be stuck with a demanding child who makes a habit of refusing food, merely to get attention.

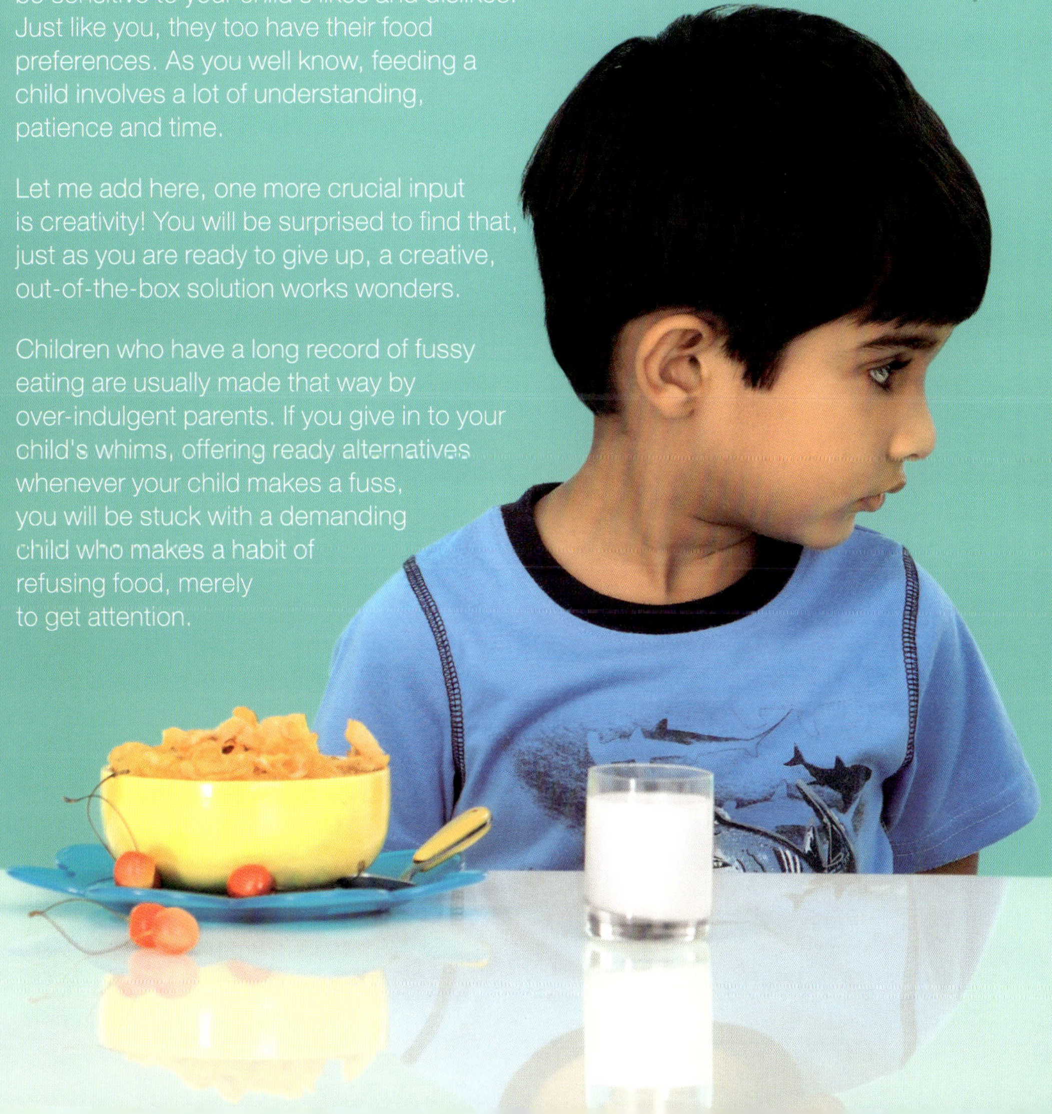

COLOUR

Different fruits and veggies are rich in different vitamins and minerals. Go for variety and pick your vegetables and fruits across the rainbow spectrum.

FACT-O-Meter

The plant kingdom offers nutrients that help prevent illness and fight disease. Each colour represents different vitamins and minerals, so eating as many colours as possible is a great way to ensure good health.

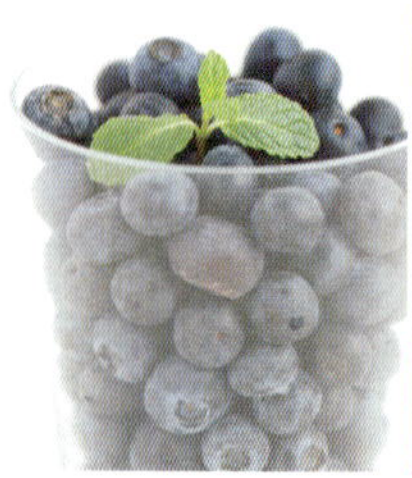
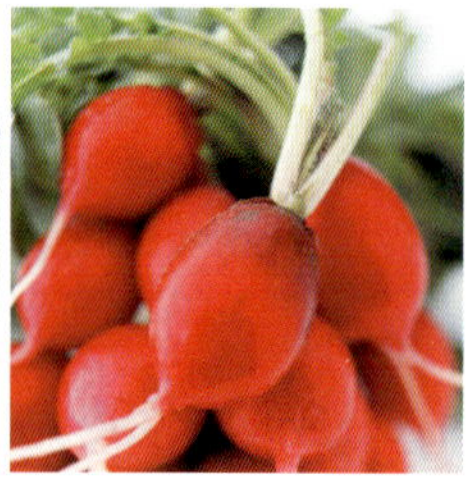
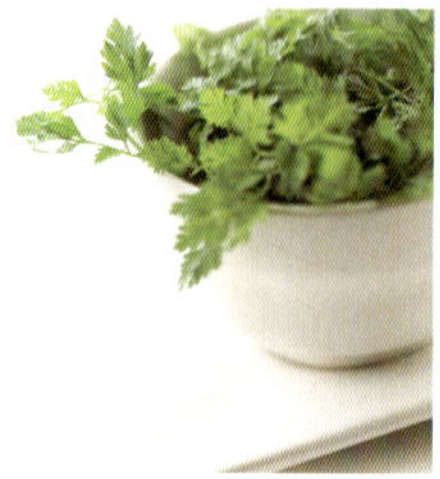

eat different colours!

Violets & Purples Beetroot contains betacyanin, an immune aid and anti-cancer agent.

Indigo Berries contain bioflavonoids that are powerful antioxidants, with health benefits that include antimicrobial, anti-inflammatory, anticancer, antihistamine and anti-allergy effects.

Blues Dark-coloured berries, grapes, contain the highest concentrations of the pigment anthocyanin, a strong antioxidant with a free radical quenching activity.

Greens Coriander, mint, asparagus, spinach, broccoli, lettuce contain chlorophyll, a protein with the same structure as hemoglobin, essential for the manufacture of red blood cells.

Yellows & Oranges Carrots, apricots, peaches, yellow peppers, squash, contain carotenoids that are good for the eyes.

Reds & Pinks Tomatoes, red peppers, grapefruit, contain lycopene, an antioxidant, which helps protect cells, maintain heart health, vision, immunity and reduce the risk of cancer.

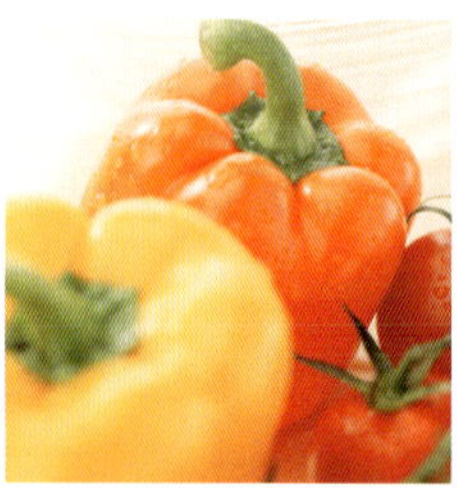
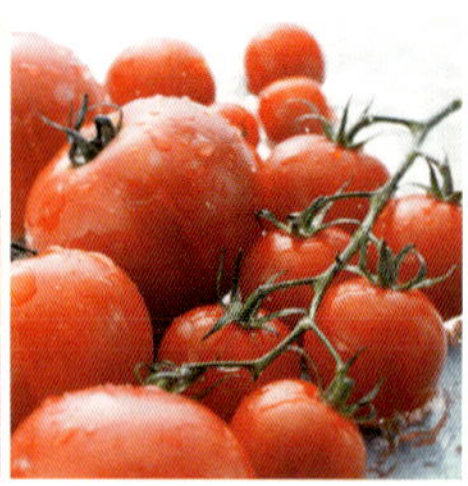
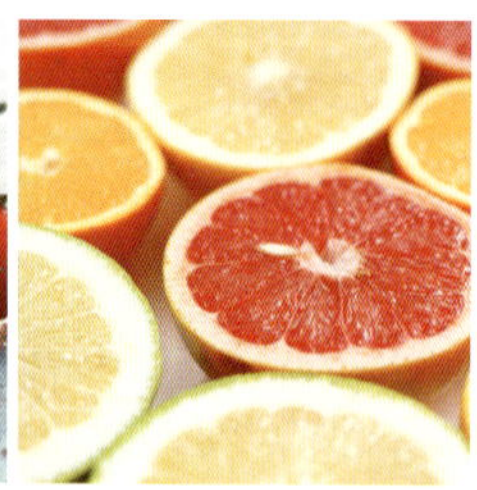

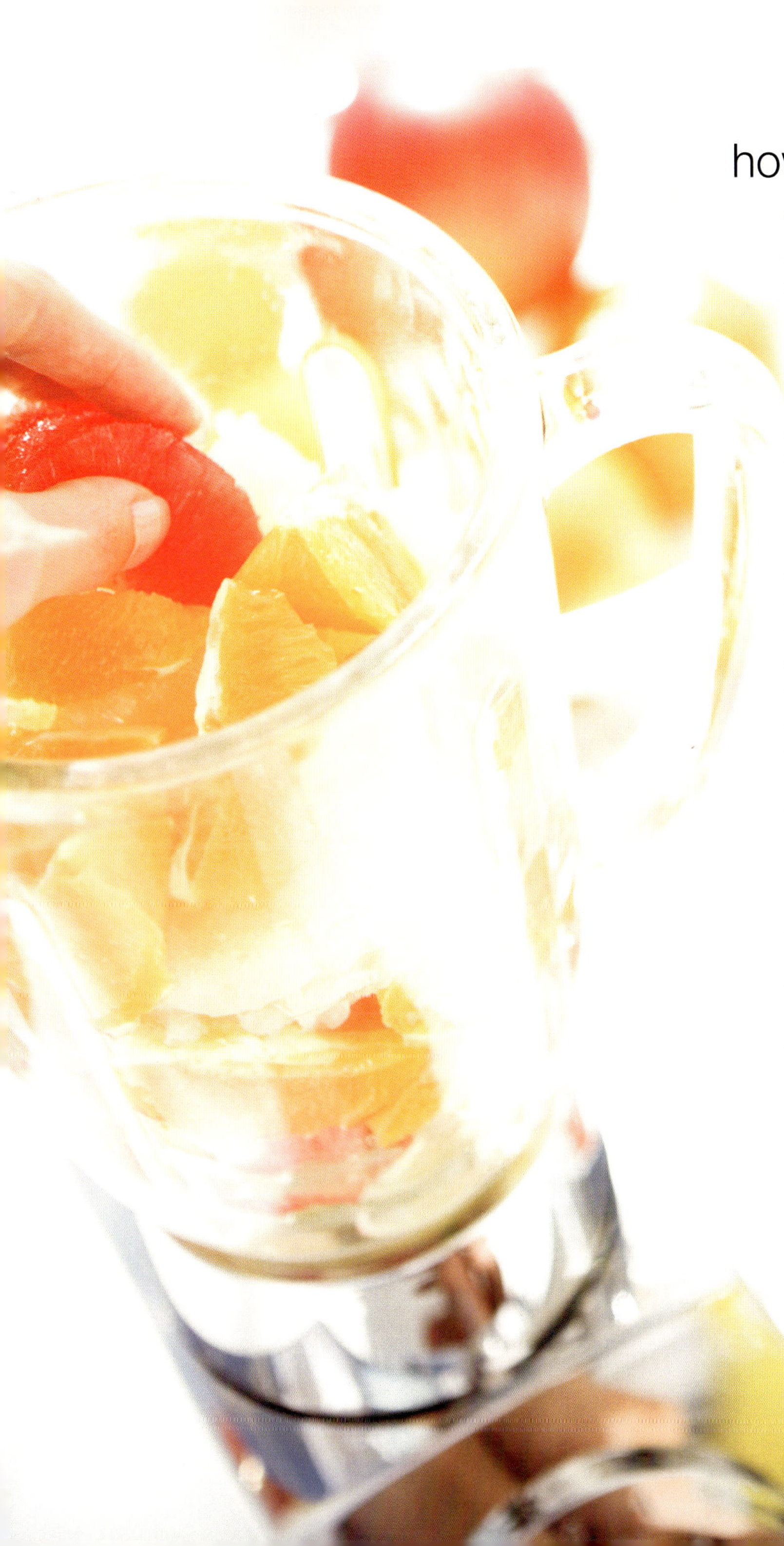

how to **TADS** it!

Transform, **A**dapt, **D**ress it Up, **S**ubstitute, or sometimes, just let it go.

For foods that remain stubbornly on your child's "yucky" list, devise alternate solutions that come with their own nutrient packed punch.

If milk is a problem, combine it into a frothy smoothie with your child's favourite fruits, or chocolate powder. If veggies are on your child's hate list, pack them into parathas, or add them, in pureed form, to dals and soups.

Make food look more appetizing. Get some cutters in different shapes, and 'design' your meal. You can cut bread, fruit, and vegetables in different shapes. Enlist your child's help, ask for an opinion in deciding colours and shapes.

HANDS-ON FUN

Children have vivid imaginations and love working with their hands. This is the perfect platform for them to unleash their kitchen skills! So team up and do something innovative, like a salad project, for example? Let your child decide a theme, you help cut, snip and curl, and lay it out.

Try baking multi-shaped cookies with a cookie cutter. Draw tomato slice faces on vegetable cutlets. Carve fruit boats with different types of melon.

The more you involve your children, the more they will enjoy and appreciate food. Take them out shopping with you, help them identify the fruits and vegetables. Let them choose what they want, even if it is not on your shopping list.

As children grow older, they need to be a part of decision–making too. Allow them to occasionally "dress" the food or help you try a new recipe.

Mayuri, who runs cookery courses today, recollects: "I love my work, thanks to Mum. I remember going to the supermarket with her every Saturday, filling in the vegetables, the fruits, the cereals, the ready-to-eats and... the packet of potato chips that I'd slyly slip in. I remember the "guess the fruit" game, or "guess the vegetable" game, which Mum and I played."

"When I grew up, I opted for a catering college course. Now I hold cookery classes and workshops. So now it is Mum's turn to, "guess the recipe" when she comes home for dinner!"

To peel or not to peel?

Does your child love crunchy apples? Juicy pears? The peel, containing 75% of the fruit's dietary fibre, is very healthy. Eating the skin of certain vegetables and fruits offers the roughage that is vital for healthy digestion. However, make sure fruits and vegetables are washed thoroughly before you let your kids get their hands on them.

shopping and stocking

Make a list of what you need. Ask your children to add to the list. Buy whole grains and dals and store healthy snacks in your pantry. Make sure to keep your refrigerator stocked with fruits, vegetables and dairy products.

Wholegrain cereals and pulses count as essentials. Fruits and vegetables are a must-have. You could either buy your produce fresh, on a daily basis or, if you can refrigerate it well, once-a-week stocking should work just fine. Milk and milk products are another all-important kitchen staple.

Non-vegetarians can freeze their poultry and seafood items in portion sized packs, for easy de-frosting.

If you have a cook at home, it is a good idea to inform him/her to be organized.

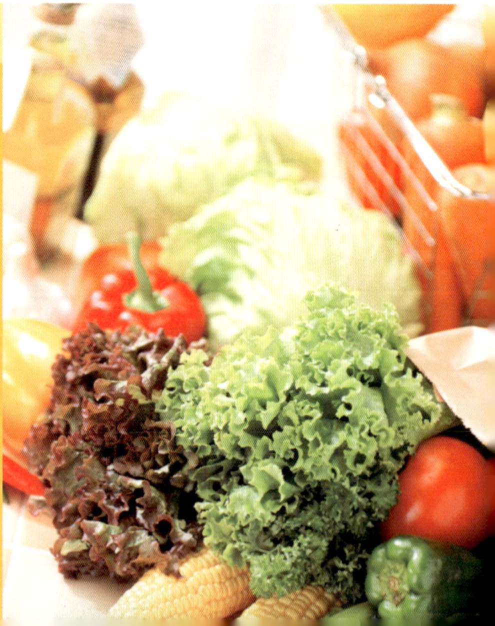

water babies

Children have small bodies that can become dehydrated very quickly. "Ma, I'm dying of thirst!" might a cry for help. Make sure your children always have access to fresh, clean drinking water. Their very survival depends on it.

FIT Alert

Be especially careful with active children, who forget to drink water or insist they are not thirsty. Children, because of their smaller size, produce more metabolic heat and therefore are more prone to dehydration than adults.

Water is one of the most essential nutrients for the human body. The adult body is 60 to 75 percent water. In children, as in adults, lack of water can cause chronic fatigue, constipation, headaches and other symptoms related to dehydration.

FACT-O-Meter

Children need 6 to 8 glasses of water every day. When they are out in hot weather, or after exercising, they need even more water to stay hydrated.

Let them have ½ a glass of water for every 30 minutes of exercise.

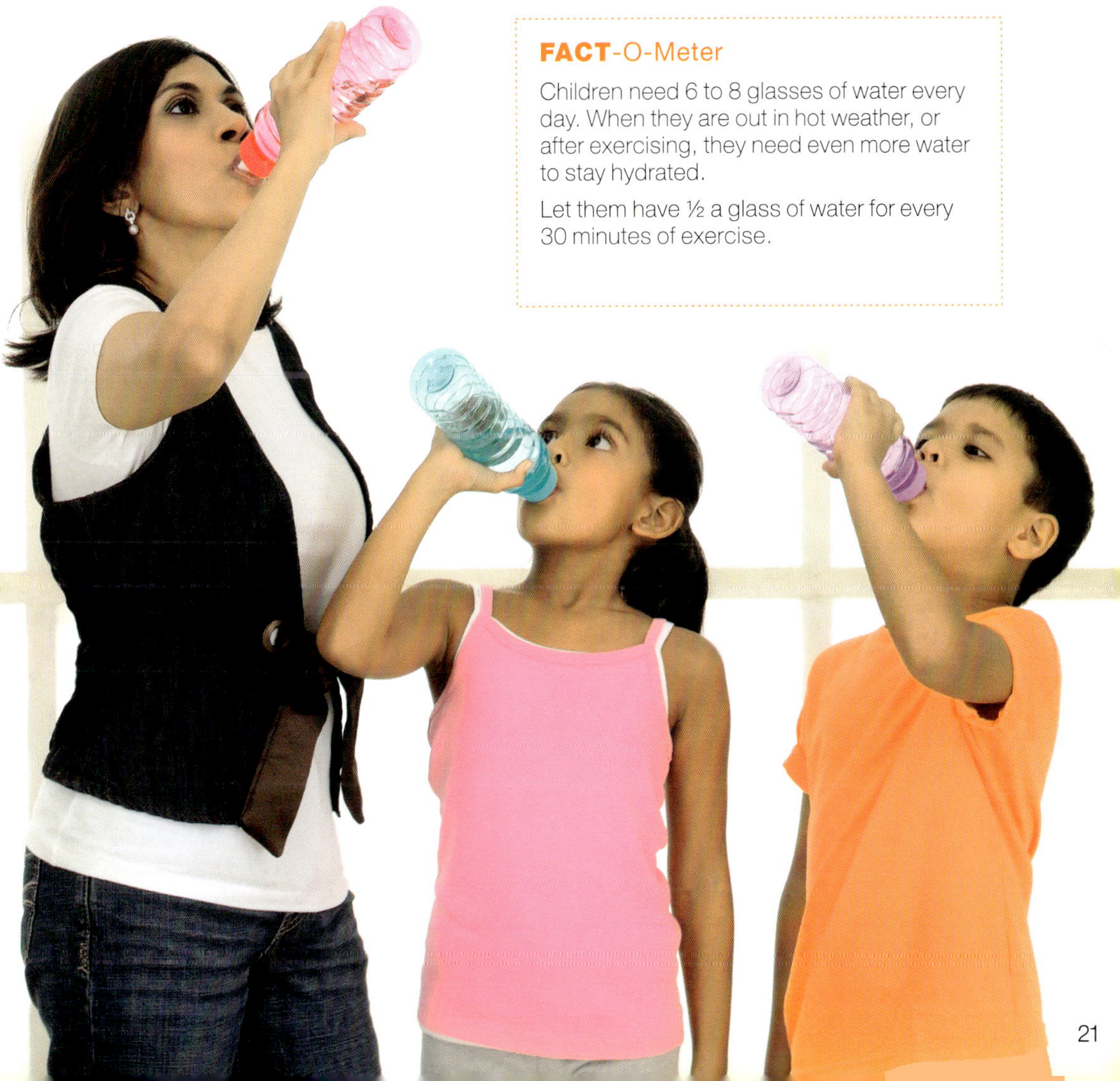

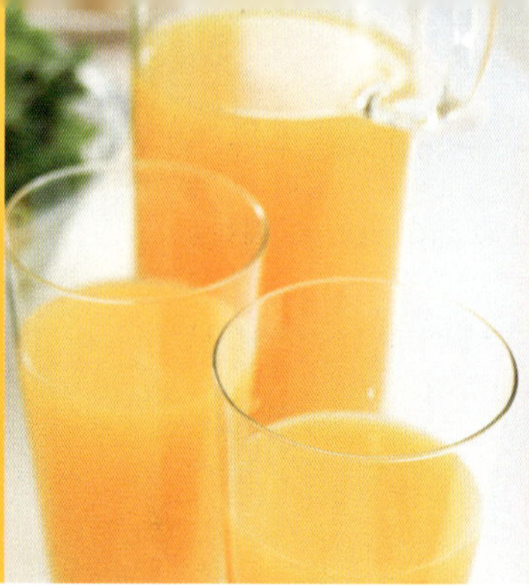

Flavoured drinks: a water substitute?

As a little kid, Radha was given an orange-flavoured squash when she got thirsty. She grew to love the colour and flavour and now, as a young adult, Radha prefers an orange soft drink over a glass of water. This acquired taste for a sweet, sugary orange drink is a childhood habit she can't seem to shake off.

On the other hand, if Radha had been encouraged to drink water from a young age, she would be more likely to stick with this habit, rather than opt for a sugary, empty calorie drink with no nutritional value whatsoever.

Q: Is it okay to drink water during meals?

A: Yes. Contrary to popular belief, water does not dilute the digestive juices. The only downside to drinking too much water with meals is that your child will feel full faster! So encourage your child to drink water only when thirsty, allowing more space for the actual meal.

Q. How do you cope with a child who has allergies? How will the child get proper nutrition?

A. Mrs. Kapoor's son, Pavan, was a happy, playful 5-year old. But milk time was tantrum time every day. At first, his mother got angry, then worried. After a medical investigation Mrs. Kapoor found that Pavan was lactose intolerant. His pediatrician suggested milk substitutes, so Pavan switched to soya milk for his protein requirement. Mrs. Kapoor was a relieved Mom, and Pavan? Growing by leaps and bounds!

food pyramid

Based on the body's nutritional needs, the food pyramid offers a balanced diet comprising the different food groups. Give your children the advantage of a varied selection of foods, from every level of the food pyramid, to ensure well-rounded nutrition for their growing needs.

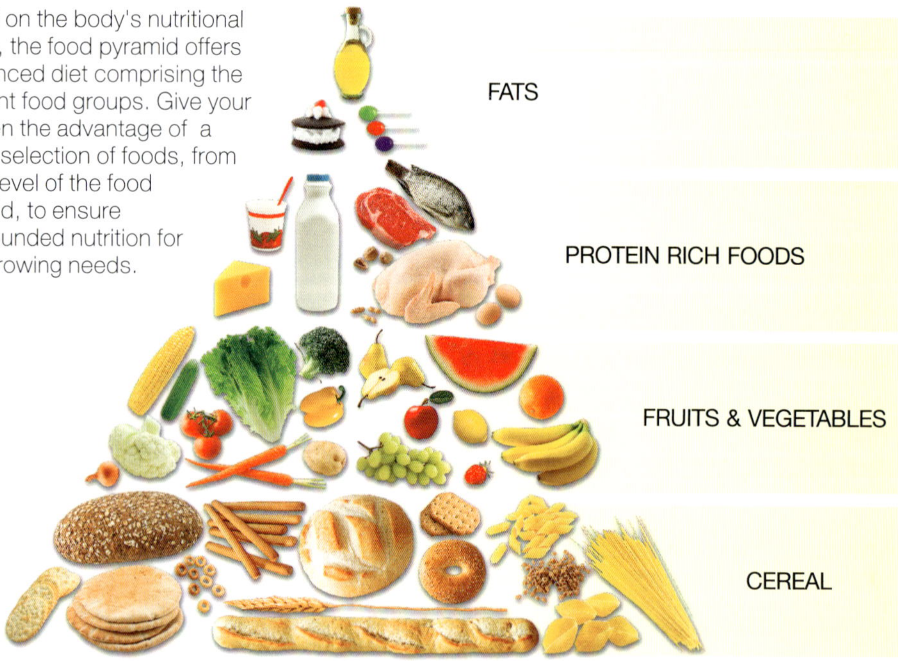

Use the food pyramid as a guide to help your family eat better every day. Each of these food groups provides some, but not all, of the nutrients needed for your child's healthy growth. No single food group is more important than the other. Each food group has its own special place on your child's plate.

However, do keep in mind, as the pyramid tapers upwards, quantities must keep decreasing.

The base of the pyramid constitutes complex carbohydrates, the bulk of a child's food requirements, eaten in the form of cereals.

The next level of the pyramid comprises fruits and vegetables, carbohydrate rich foods that are loaded with vitamins and minerals.

The third level of the pyramid represents proteins. The body requires fewer servings of protein than carbohydrates.

At the tip, the fourth level, are fats, oils and sweets, to be consumed in small amounts.

CEREAL: For a power-packed performance

This category includes grains like rice, wheat, barley, jowar, ragi and oats. Grain variants such as poha, sooji, oatmeal, kurmura and pasta also count as cereals. All cereals contain carbohydrates, for that great boost of energy, vital for active kids of every age.

Try to make wholegrain choices instead of consuming refined products like maida. This is because whole grains keep the original nutrients intact. They also retain all the natural fibre. Powerhouse wholegrain options are red rice, bajra, ragi, dahlia and oats.

FIT Tips

Read the labels of products and lookout for words like "wholegrain" or "unpolished". When you cook rice, do not drain out the excess water, because you lose precious vitamins in the water that is thrown away.

FACT-O-Meter

Refined grains are prepared by milling. The bran and germ layer of the grain is removed. This reduces fibre content, folic acid, selenium, vitamin E and many other valuable nutrients.

FRUITS & VEGETABLES: Naturally the best

Experiment with nature's bounty! Your child's fruit and veggie intake can be in the form of fresh, uncooked veggies, like salads, or you could opt for lightly cooked vegetables. Over-cooking or boiling vegetables destroys their vitamins and minerals, so make sure veggies are steamed or lightly sautéed, giving your child the full benefit of what nature has to offer.

Myth: Tinned or frozen fruit and vegetables aren't healthy

FACT: Fresh is always best, provided it is consumed fresh. Today, frozen or canned fruits and vegetables are just as nutritious as the fresh version, because produce is packed within hours of being picked. Modern processing and packing techniques allow nutrients to be better retained in the freezing or canning process.

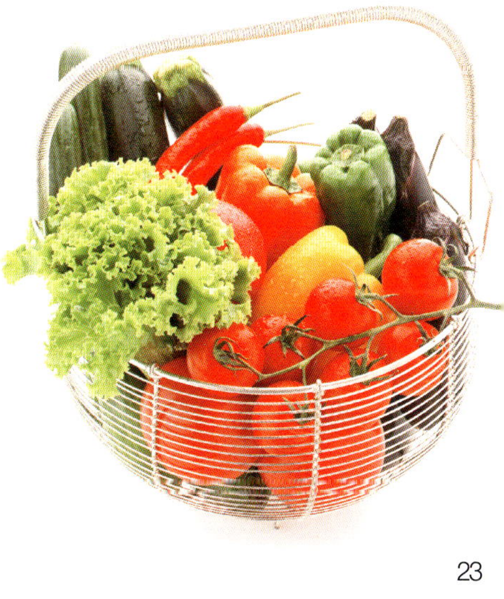

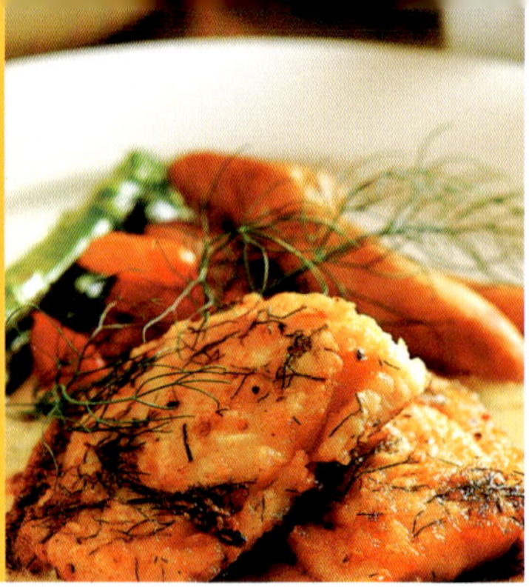

PROTEIN-RICH FOODS: For children's growing needs

Proteins work to repair and regenerate muscle tissue and are known as the body's building blocks. The body breaks protein down into amino acids, which are used to build and maintain muscles, bones, body organs, the blood and the immune system. Pulses, dairy products, fish and chicken, sprouts and seeds, all have high protein value.

In the Indian diet, pulses and dairy products are the primary source of protein for vegetarians.

Non-vegetarians are assured better health benefits when fish is eaten boiled, baked, grilled, or steamed. Frying the fish alters its fatty acid composition, destroying its beneficial effects.

FACT-O-Meter

How much protein does your child need? The formula is approximately 1 gram of protein for every kilogram of bodyweight. So if a child weighs, say 25 kilos, the protein requirement is 25 grams per day.

Q. Are vegetarian diets protein deficient?

A. No. Vegetarians get their full protein supply from pulses and grains, milk and milk products and soya products. Animal sources such as milk and milk products are complete sources of protein. Vegetable proteins are incomplete and need to be combined with other foods to be complete.

For example, grains combined with lentil, like dal and roti, or nuts and seeds with grain, are excellent sources of complete vegetarian protein.

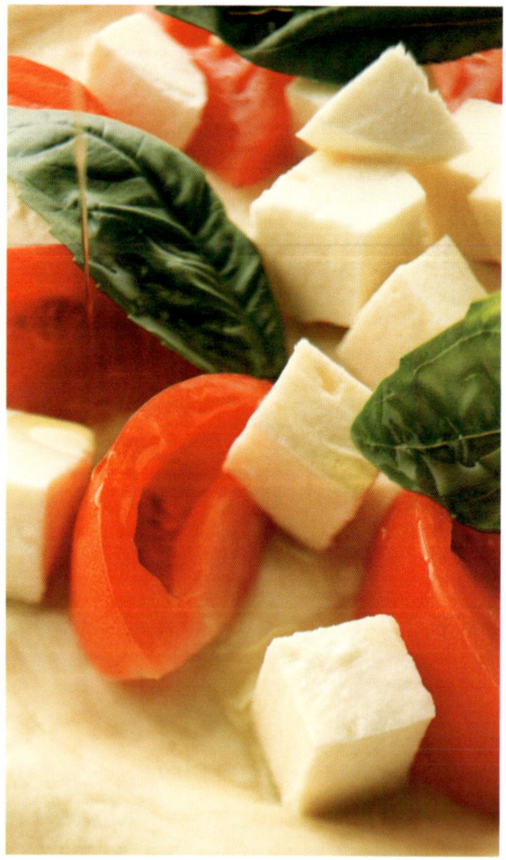

All the vegetarian items in the following list provide protein value of approximately 7 grams. This protein content is the same as 30 grams of meat.

- ¼ cup cottage cheese
- 240 ml milk (8 grams protein)
- ½ cup cooked legumes or lentil
- ⅓ cup curd
- ¼ cup tofu
- 1 cup soy milk
- 2 tablespoons mixed nuts

FATS: An essential addition

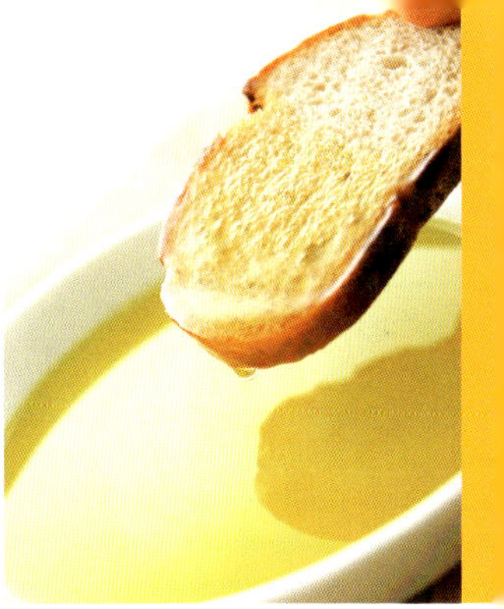

An adequate fat intake is essential for growth and development. Fats are needed to build cells, provide energy, preserve body heat and protect organs from damage. Vitamins A, D, E and K require fat in order to be absorbed. These vitamins help in hormone production and are necessary for insulating all nervous system tissue in the body.

Let's understand that "adequate" fat does not mean unlimited fat. A small amount is all that is required to meet your child's nutritional needs. Too much fat can lead to obesity and ill-health.

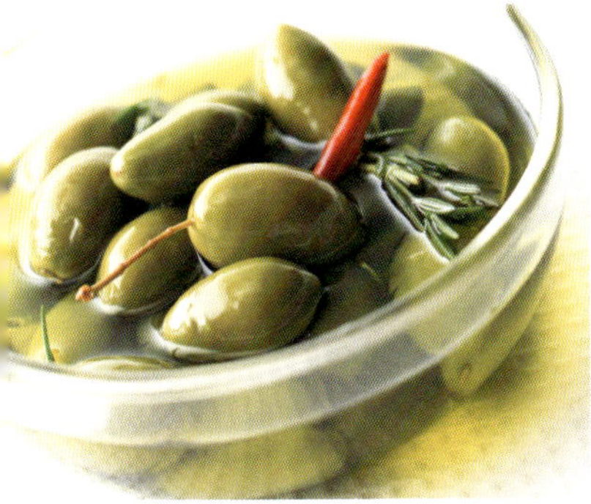

What are good fats, and why are they good?

Examples of good fats are monounsaturated fats like olive, peanut and canola oil. Polyunsaturated fats, from plant sources such as corn and sunflower, are also considered beneficial. These are aii considered good fats because, when consumed in small quantities, they reduce blood cholesterol and protect against heart disease.

Ayurveda encourages the consumption of ghee. In India, traditional cooking methods make use of ghee and fresh butter.

your child's daily nutrition chart

CARBOHYDRATE	(4 - 8 years)	170 - 250 grams
	(9 -14 years)	300 grams
PROTEINS	(4 - 8 years)	18 28 grams
	(9 -14 years)	28 - 50 grams
FATS	(4 - 8 years)	40 - 60 grams
	(9 -14 years)	60 -75 grams
Total daily calories	(4 - 8 years)	1500 - 2000 calories
	(9 -14 years)	1800 - 2200 calories

Getting into a healthy eating pattern is not difficult. A little bit of effort to change your children's eating patterns can make a substantial difference to their well-being!

Please check my website www.liveactive.com for more detailed information on nutrition.

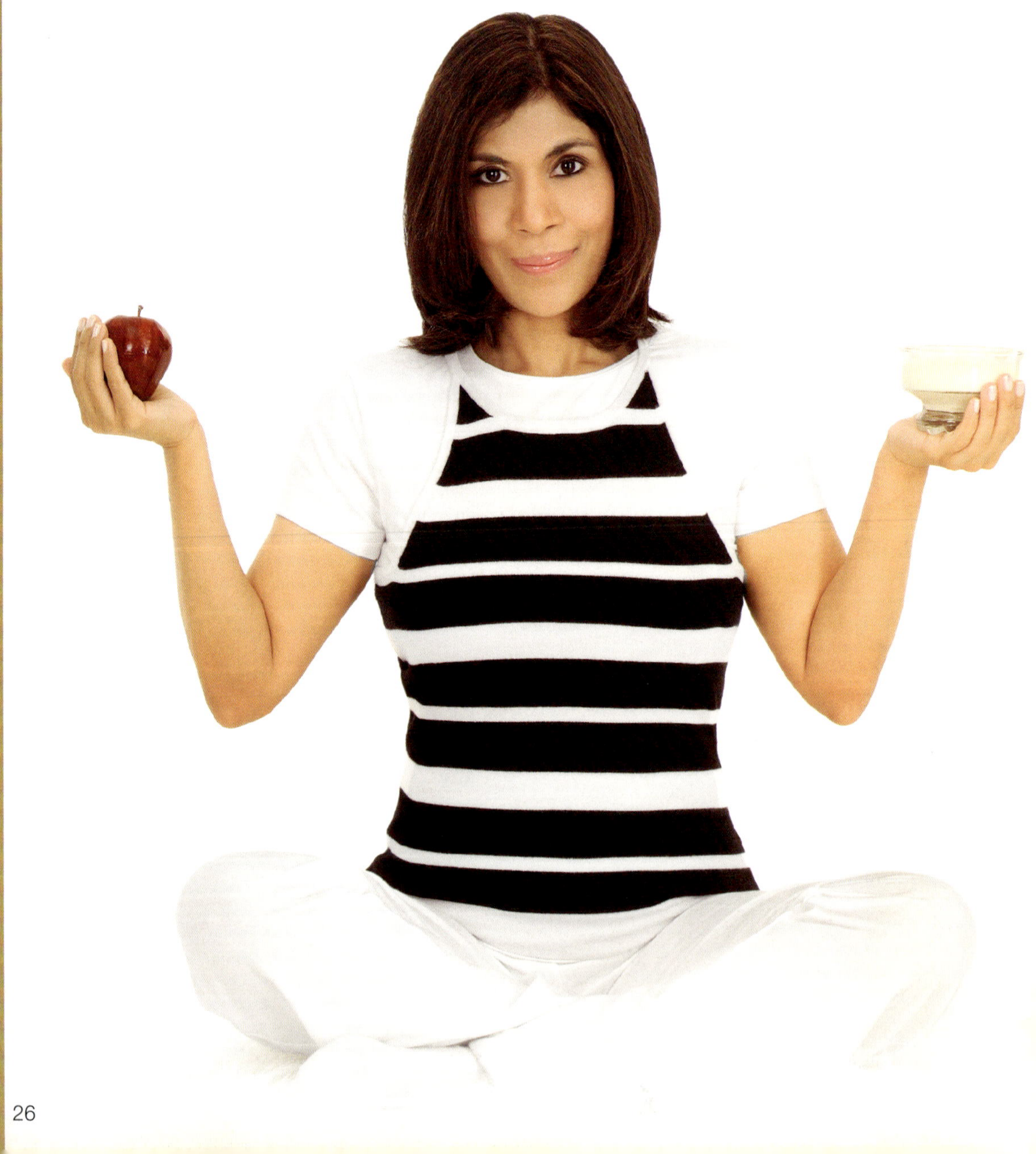

Mantra 2

Childhood needs are **unique,** requiring unique nutrition. A **healthy diet** is integral for growing **bones,** developing **minds,** extra **energy** reserves, a sound **digestive system** and enhanced **immunity.**

FOOD INSURANCE POLICY

When you are looking at raising a healthy, well-rounded child, you wonder how best to ensure adequate nutrition. So many questions pop up. Should kids have extra calcium or vitamin supplements? Do they need more protein as they grow? How much fat can they consume?

What your child eats determines how your child grows. Kids must have a varied diet, to take care of their unique needs. Their bones are growing. Their minds are developing. Their bodies need surplus energy. Their digestive systems require care. Last but not least, immunity also has to be built up, to protect children against infection.

Sounds like a tall order, doesn't it? Don't fret too much, because realistically speaking, if your children eat well and maintain regular meal times, you have them insured on all counts. In the previous chapter, Mantra 1, I have detailed what a balanced meal should look like. It is important to offer a balanced food plan, with an emphasis on forming healthy food habits. This is the best insurance plan you can give your children – for life!

For more information on the right food choices, please log onto my website www.liveactive.com

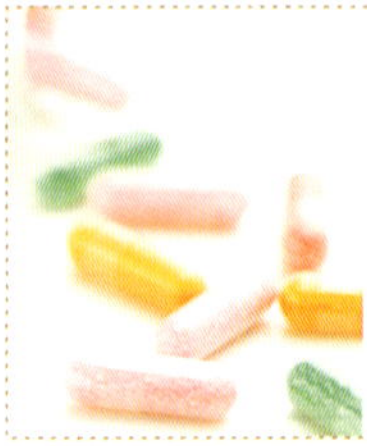

Q: Are vitamin supplements necessary for a child's health?

A: A balanced diet provides the body with the necessary vitamins and minerals. Extra supplements should always be prescribed by your child's physician, based on individual needs and concerns.

food for the bones

CALCIUM, A SECURITY DEPOSIT FOR YOUR CHILD'S BONES

There is more calcium in the human body than any other mineral. The maximum amount of calcium, about 99%, is found deposited in the teeth and bones. The remaining 1% is found in soft tissue.

Apart from calcium intake, weight bearing exercises are a crucial input for bone strength. Walking, running, jumping, and outdoor games are examples of weight bearing activities. During childhood and through adolescence, these activities enhance bone strength and density, by increasing calcium deposits in the bones. Regular exercise in childhood also reduces the risk of ailments such as osteoporosis, which are common in later stages of life.

FIT Alert!
Studies show that very often, children, especially in the 11-14 age group, fail to get their recommended daily calcium requirement. Girls of this age tend to avoid dairy foods which are a rich source of calcium, on the grounds that milk and milk products are fattening.

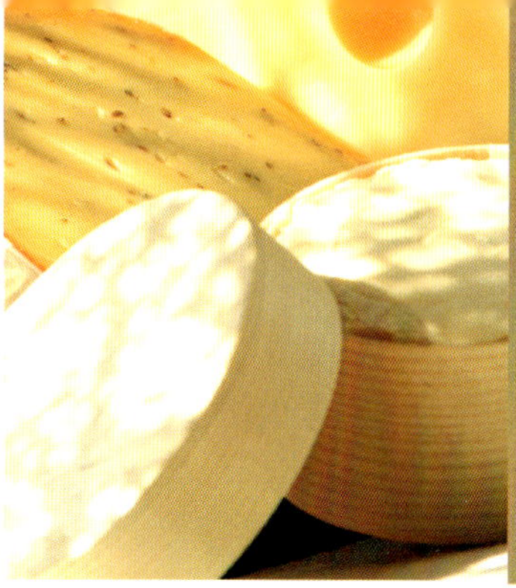

Calcium-rich foods

Milk, yoghurt, orange juice, almonds, cheese, sardines, oysters, green vegetables, beans and broccoli.

Did you know ?

The human skeleton is made up of 206 bones, giving the body its basic framework. The process of bone development continues through childhood and adolescence. Bone growth is rapid during the crucial years of 4 to 14.

The sunshine vitamin

Vitamin D is called the "sunshine vitamin" because it is made when sunlight touches the skin! The early morning rays of the sun are gentle and will provide your child with valuable vitamin D, required for the absorption of calcium into the system. A deficiency in vitamin D can lead to unsatisfactory bone growth in children.

Foods containing Vitamin D

Milk, egg yolk, tuna and salmon.

FACT-O-Meter

Children who drink fizzy or caffeinated beverages get less calcium because these substances inhibit the body's absorption of calcium.

CALCIUM BOOSTER - COTTAGE CHEESE SPREAD

Nutrients : calcium, vitamins A, B12, D, iron, magnesium, phosphorus

Preparation time : 10 minutes

Serves : 2

Ingredients : ½ cup crumbled low fat cottage cheese / paneer
2 tablespoons yoghurt, hung
2 tablespoons chopped coriander
¼ teaspoon crushed garlic, optional
½ tablespoon chopped spring onions, optional
salt to taste
1 tablespoon toasted sesame seeds

Directions : Mix the ingredients. Spread on wholegrain bread, crackers, or use as a dip.

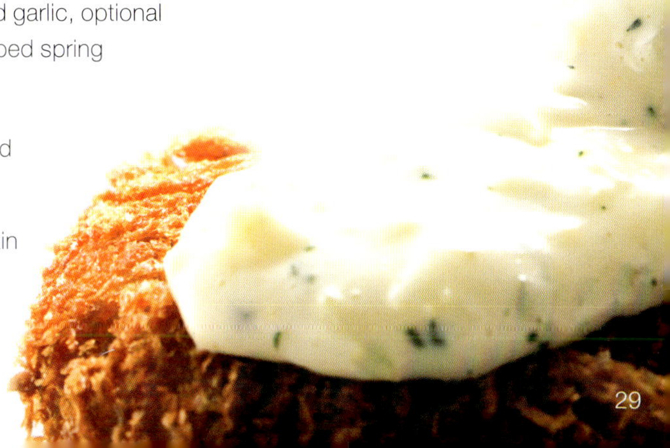

food for the mind

When your daughter has had too much candy, or has skipped a meal, you will find she tends to get irritable. Food affects the brain in many different ways. The brain uses ingredients from the food your child eats, to manufacture brain chemicals, essential for helping children to think, learn, play a sport, sing, dance and much more.

Simply put, the brain likes a steady supply of nutrients, and dislikes extreme fluctuations. The ups and downs of blood sugar can create a neurotransmitter imbalance, causing your child to feel fidgety, irritable, inattentive and even sleepy.

The process of brain growth is dynamic and lifelong. There is a direct co-relation between your child's learning environment, individual capacity, and the nutrients your child consumes. Remember, optimum nutrition is a huge factor in sharpening the mind and improving memory. Omega 3 and omega 6 fatty acids contribute to optimum brain performance. Fish, shellfish, nuts, seeds and oils from soya bean, safflower, flax seeds and walnuts contain high levels of omega-3 and omega-6 fatty acids.

FACT-O-Meter

More than 60% of the brain is composed of fat. Fats regulate key aspects of memory and mood. Lack of essential fats in your child's diet can lead to poor memory.

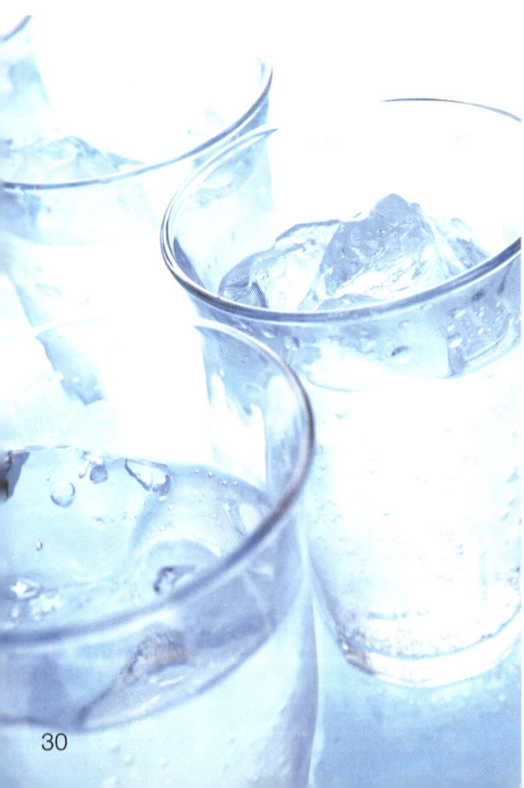

5 SECRETS FOR A HEALTHY MIND

1. Engage in active learning throughout life.
2. Interact with people and lead an active social life.
3. Sleep well. 7 to 9 hours of sleep is essential, so make sure you get a good night's sleep.
4. Have a positive attitude. A positive spirit ensures not only a healthy mind but also a healthy heart.
5. Drink at least 8 glasses of water every day, to hydrate brain cells.

Water constitutes about 83% of total blood composition. Within the body, blood acts as a transport system, delivering nutrients to the brain and eliminating toxins. Dehydration results in fatigue and diminished concentration levels.

Give your children colourful straws to sip water, or a glass with cartoon characters, floral designs, or even a personalized logo – this makes drinking water fun!

Nuts over nuts

We tend to think of nuts as snack foods, but seldom stop to consider their nutritional benefits. Nuts are terrific sources of healthy oils, especially vitamin E. The protein in nuts is important for growth and repair of tissues, and the fat provides the body essential fatty acids, vital to good health. Once your children start eating nuts, it's hard to stop them! Nuts should be eaten in limited quantities, as they contain a high percentage of fat.

TIP

A handful is enough, a bowlful is not required! Just 5-6 almonds a day will help to boost memory.

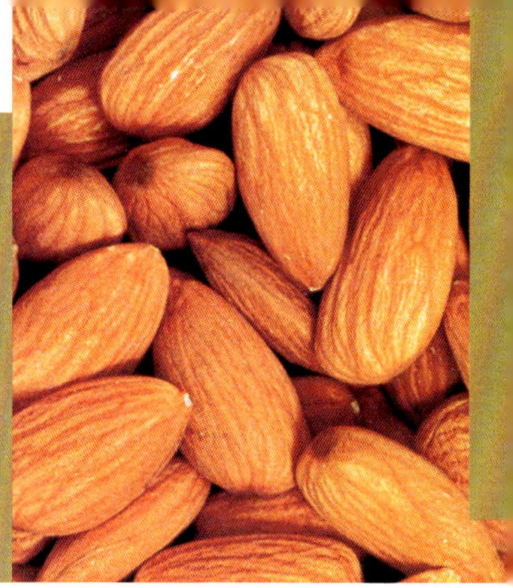

CHIKKI RECIPE

Nutrients	:	vitamins E, B1, B2, B3, calcium, copper, magnesium, manganese, iron, selenium, zinc, protein, calcium
Preparation time	:	10 minutes
Serves	:	10 pieces
Ingredients	:	½ cup puffed rice ½ cup sesame seeds sunflower seeds chopped mixed nuts ½ cup jaggery
Directions	:	Heat the jaggery on a low flame until it melts. Add the roasted puffed rice, sesame and sunflower seeds, nuts, and mix well. Pour this mixture onto a smooth stone surface. Roll into a sheet using a rolling pin. Cut into pieces. Store in an airtight container.

food for energy

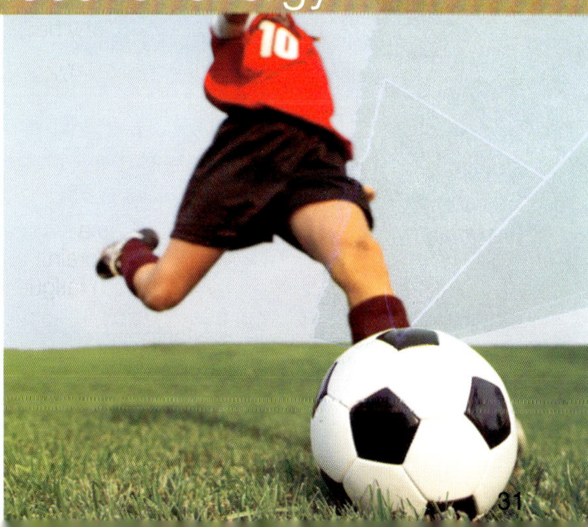

Topping up the energy levels

Just looking at your energetic kid can make you feel tired! Chasing young children takes up so much of your energy, you can imagine how much fuel they need to keep that energy topped up. Younger kids are always on the move, running, playing, jumping, climbing. Even older kids, with their love for sports and the outdoor life, expend huge amounts of energy.

Q: My son Mehul, a 12-year old, is a keen swimmer. He comes home famished after his swim. What can I give him?

A: When children are actively involved in sports you need to monitor their diet closely and carefully. See that your kid does not skip breakfast and gets enough energy boosters through the day. Regular, balanced meals are very important, offered in adequate amounts, at frequent intervals.

FIT Facts

Protein and carb combo snacks are great energy providers.

Give your child cereal and yoghurt, a piece of toasted wholegrain bread with an egg, or a peanut butter sandwich as fuel after activity.

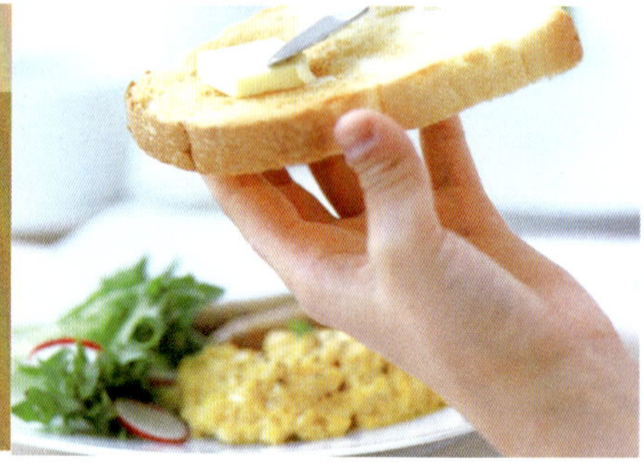

Whey protein

Whey is the watery liquid which is left over after making cottage cheese. It contains lactic acid, as well as valuable proteins, which help for better digestion. When you make paneer, do not discard the whey. Add it to soups, or mix it in chapatti dough for added nutrition.

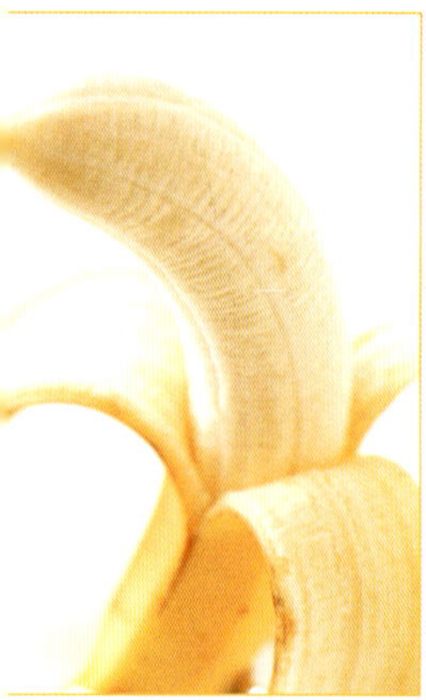

That extra kick!

Rikin and Nikhil are football buddies. They go for football coaching five times a week after school and come home ravenous and exhausted. Rikin's Mum has a banana and a cup of yoghurt ready for him after play. Bananas give him instant energy and Rikin enjoys dipping them in flavoured yoghurt.

Nikhil, on the other hand, ate a packet of chips and candy after play. His energy levels dipped and he continued to feel tired. A couple of times, when Nikhil came to Rinkin's after a game, Rikin's Mum offered both the boys a healthy snack. Nikhil felt the difference, and, on returning home, he informed his Mom that he too wanted to snack healthy!

After Nikhil switched to protein-carb combo snacks, the "washed out" feeling became a thing of the past, much to his mother's relief.

FIT Alert

Deficiency in calcium and iron can hinder athletic performance. Calcium is vital for athletes whose bodies have to endure stress, and require strong, healthy bones to perform well. Similarly, an iron deficiency can cause early fatigue, thereby lowering performance.

BANANA-NUT SPREAD

Nutrients : calcium, vitamins A, B12, D, iron, magnesium, phosphorus

Preparation time : 5 minutes

Serves : 2

Ingredients : 1 banana, peeled and mashed with a fork

1 teaspoon raisins

1 teaspoon chopped dates

1 teaspoon chopped nuts (almonds, walnuts and cashew nuts)

Directions : Mix the ingredients and use as topping on wholegrain bread or crackers.

SMOOTHIE

Nutrients : vitamins B3, B5, B6, B12, C, E, biotin, magnesium, manganese, potassium, fibre, calcium, phosphorous, zinc, iron

Preparation time : 5 minutes

Serves : 2

Ingredients : 2 small bananas, chopped

1 cup milk

¼ glass water

1 tablespoon powdered almonds

2 teaspoons honey

Directions : Put the bananas, milk, water and powdered almonds in a blender. Add the honey and buzz again until smooth and frothy.

food for digestion

'You are what you eat' is only partially true. You are also what you digest and absorb. The ability to digest well is therefore vital for your child's physical and mental well being.

Mona, an 8-year old, was bad-tempered on school mornings and always late for the school bus. Her mother realized that her daughter was constipated. Mona's problem was, she had to rush through her morning routine, to make it to the school in time.

A friend suggested Mona be given 4-5 prunes, or dried figs soaked in water, as a daily snack. Her mother also made sure that Mona woke up slightly earlier in the mornings, so that she had time to eat her breakfast.

It was an effort for Mona to get accustomed to the new routine, but thankfully, she did. A few days later, as she queued up for her school bus, friends noticed how happy and cheerful Mona had become!

FACT-O-Meter

It is important to chew every bite of food 20 times. Teeth are designed to grind food to a liquid mush and the saliva begins the digestive process in the mouth itself. When your child eats too fast, food is semi-digested, and its full nutritional value is lost.

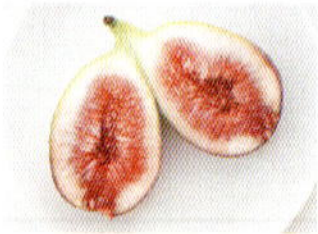

1. Figs / Prunes / Raisins
   Figs, prunes and raisins improve digestion and elimination. Rich in iron and calcium, they also improve blood quality and build strong bones.

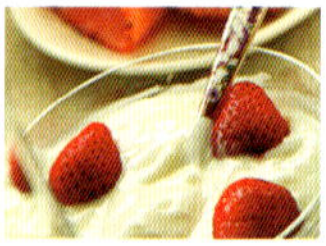

2. Yoghurt
   Yoghurt contains probiotics which are responsible for several activities in the gut, such as producing lactase, killing harmful bacteria and improving digestive tract function. Probiotics are the friendly bacteria found in the gut, helping to build immunity.

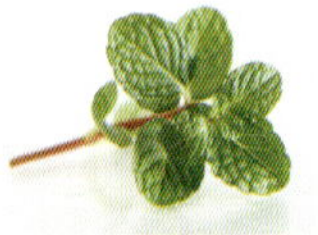

3. Mint
   Mint is used to treat flatulence and indigestion. It can also stimulate the appetite and cure nausea and headaches. Peppermint tea can help soothe a dry throat.

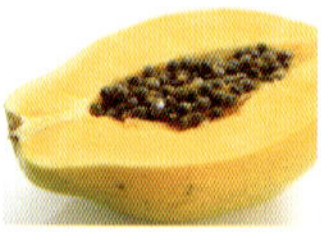

4. Papaya
   Papaya contains the enzyme papain, which improves digestion. It reduces the risk of heart disease and promotes digestive health.

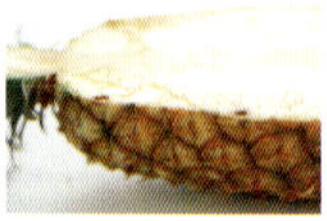

5. Pineapple
   Pineapple is a diuretic, which detoxifies the body. It contains the enzyme bromelin, which improves digestive functioning.

FIBRE: The body's internal broom

As fibre passes through the digestive tract, it acts like a sponge, cleaning out waste matter and preventing constipation.

Once upon a time, it was called "roughage," a term grandmothers still use. But the advice to eat more roughage is still up-to-date! Give your child fibre-rich foods like whole grains, lentils, nuts, beans, seeds, and plenty of fruits and vegetables. Avoid, as much as possible, processed foods and foods containing artificial additives.

FIT Tip

When you increase your child's fibre intake, it is necessary to increase water and fluid intake as well. Fibre binds with water, adding bulk and softness to the stool and regularizing bowel movement. Transit time within the intestinal tract is also accelerated, thereby eliminating waste at a faster rate.

FIBRE CONTENT OF SOME FOODS

FOOD GROUP	QUANTITY	GRAMS OF FIBRE
Beans and lentils		
Lentils cooked	½ cup	7.8
Kidney beans cooked	½ cup	7.3
Chickpeas cooked	½ cup	5.3
Cereals		
Oatmeal cooked	1 cup	4
Raisin bran	¾ cup	5
Breads and grains		
Brown rice cooked	½ cup	2
Whole-wheat bread	1 slice	2
Fruits		
Pear with skin	1	4
Apple with skin	1	3.7
Peach with skin	1	3.4
Figs dried	2	4
Vegetables		
Carrot	1	2
Tomato	1	2
Broccoli cooked	½ cup	2
Spinach cooked	½ cup	2

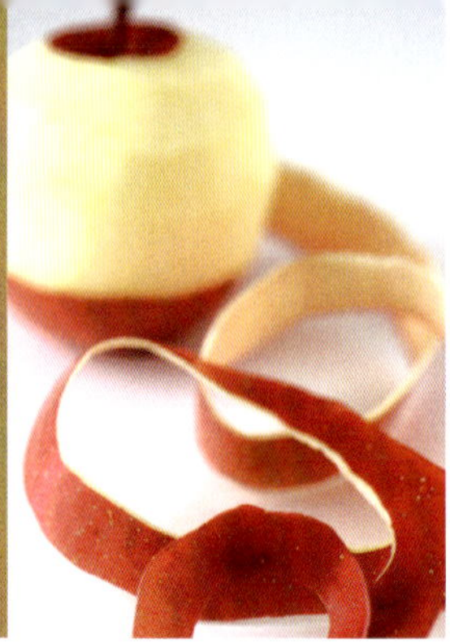

5 SECRETS TO GET MORE FIBRE

1. Add atta instead of maida, to thicken soups, pasta sauce and gravies.
2. Eat the skin of the fruit (after thorough washing).
3. Offer a handful of mixed nuts when kids feel "snacky".
4. Try bajra, ragi, brown rice, oatmeal as cereal options to whole wheat.
5. Give coconut water straight from the shell, with fun straws for sipping.

food for immunity

My neighbour Mrs. Mehta insisted that her 7-year old Divesh was always the 'first to catch flu'. Our conversations in the elevator centred around leaky noses, ear aches, stomach upsets, and bouts of fever! I explained to her that germs are part of a child's world. Kids are exposed to bacteria, viruses, fungi and parasites, and you cannot 'germ proof' a child.

Immunity is a combined function of the lymphatic system, the bloodstream, the digestive system and the skin, all working in combat mode to defend the body from invaders.

Immunity boosters

- good hygiene
  make sure your children wash their hands after returning from school or from the playground.
- the sleep fortifier
  lack of sleep reduces immunity. So make sure your child gets 8 to10 hours of sleep every day.
- laugh and hug your child to good health
  believe it or not, a regular dose of hugs and kisses keeps the bugs at bay. Studies show that laughter and positive thinking boost immunity. Stress and unhappiness lower a child's resistance to disease. The more children laugh and enjoy life, the better their immune function.
- a balanced, well-planned diet
  include foods with vitamin C, zinc, iron
- good digestive health
- regular exercise
- positive attitude

Immunity downers

- stress
- improper diet
- sedentary habits
- inadequate rest and sleep
- pesticides
- food additives
- pollution

For more information on the various subjects covered here, visit my website at www.liveactive.com

VITAL VITAMINS AND MINERALS

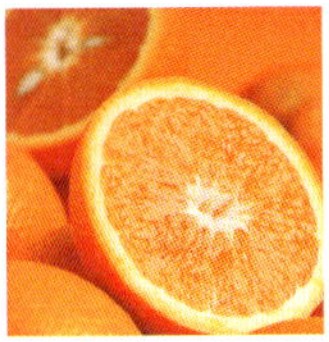

1. Vitamin C

   All immune system organs and cells rely on specific nutrients to function efficiently. For example, interferon, an anti-viral and anti cancer chemical, secreted by tissues throughout the body, needs vitamin C for its production. Fruits, vegetables, whole grains, seeds and sprouts are a rich source of antioxidant vitamin C.

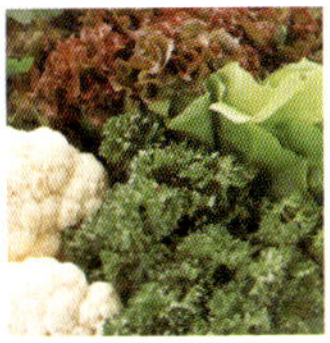

2. Iron

   If your child is tired and low on energy, it could be the sign of an iron deficiency. Iron increases hemoglobin in the blood, so a drop in hemoglobin levels can lead to anemia and fatigue. Green leafy vegetables, beans and meat are good sources of iron.

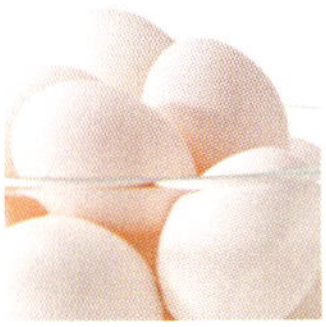

3. Zinc

   Zinc is necessary for cell division, growth and wound healing. Almost every cell in the body contains zinc. Adequate levels of zinc are vital to health and a deficiency can cause loss of appetite and reduced resistance to infection. Eggs, milk, whole wheat foods, grains and peanuts are good sources of zinc.

IMMUNITY-BOOSTING HIGH-FIBRE CHUTNEY

Nutrients : iron, magnesium, phosphorus, vitamin B6, selenium, amino acids, vitamins C & E

Preparation time : 5 minutes

Serves : ½ cup

Ingredients : 1 cup coriander and mint, washed and finely chopped
2 teaspoons jaggery (crumbled)
¼ cup fresh green garlic, chopped
1 teaspoon lemon juice
½ teaspoon ginger, crushed
salt to taste

Directions : Grind all the ingredients in a food processor, using approximately 2 tablespoons water. Enjoy as an accompaniment to snacks, or spread in sandwiches.

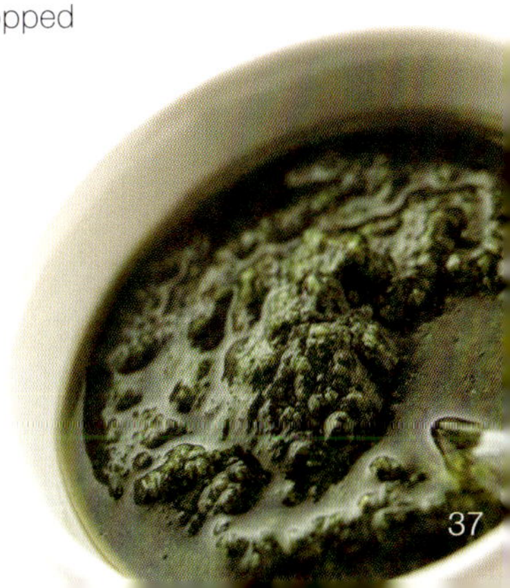

THE A, B, C OF VITAMINS & MINERALS

Vitamins & minerals	What it Does	Best Food Sources	Signs Of Deficiency
Vitamin A	maintains healthy eyes, skin, antioxidant, protects against infections and cancer	carrots, cabbage, pumpkin, sweet potato, broccoli, liver, eggs, melon, apricots, papaya, spinach, milk	poor night vision, dry flaky skin, frequent colds, acne
Vitamin C	strengthens immune system, absorbs iron, heals wounds, fights infection	citrus fruits, tomatoes, strawberries, cabbage, broccoli, melon	frequent colds & infection, easy bruising, nose bleeds, tender gums
Vitamin B12	formation of red blood cells	oysters, tuna, eggs, cottage cheese, cheese, milk, chicken	lack of energy, constipation, tender muscles, pale skin, irritability
Vitamin D	essential for bone growth & calcium absorption	dairy products, fish, egg yolks, sunlight	tooth decay, weak bones, hair loss
Vitamin K	helps to clot the blood	leafy green vegetables, cauliflower, fruit	
Vitamin E	for blood functioning & fighting of free radicals	vegetable oils & eggs	
Folic Acid	helps body use proteins, promotes formation of red blood cells	nuts, whole grains, leafy green vegetables, citrus fruits	anemia, anxiety, lack of energy, poor appetite
Calcium	promotes a healthy heart, healthy nerves, improves skin, bones, teeth	cheese, almonds, prunes, dried beans, cabbage, pumpkin seeds, dairy products	muscle cramps, tooth decay, nervousness
Potassium	maintains fluid balance in the body, stimulates gut movements, helps secretion of insulin	radish, pumpkin, cauliflower, cabbage, potatoes with skin, bananas, dried fruits, pulses, leafy vegetables	nausea, diarrhoea, muscle weakness, irritability

Vitamins & Minerals	What it Does	Best Food Sources	Signs Of Deficiency
Magnesium	strengthens bones and teeth, promotes healthy muscles	wheat germ, almonds, cashew nuts, peanuts, garlic, raisins, green peas, potato skin	muscle weakness, lack of appetite, nervousness
Iron	forms haemoglobin, vital for producing red blood cells	leafy green vegetables, pulses, whole grains, dried fruits, egg yolk, salmon	anemia, pale skin, fatigue, loss of appetite
Zinc	promotes cell growth, bone & tooth formation, heals wounds	peanuts, pulses, egg yolks, whole wheat	greasy skin, acne, loss of appetite, frequent infection

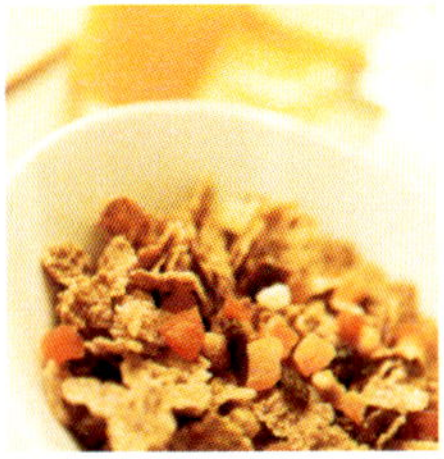

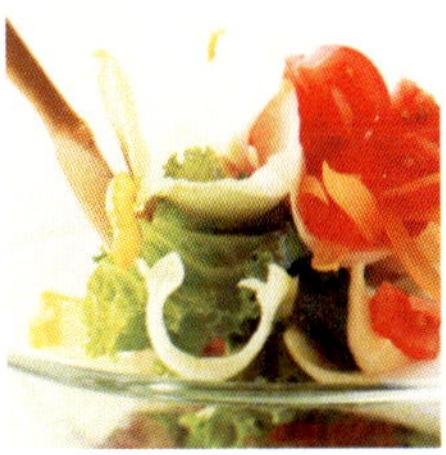

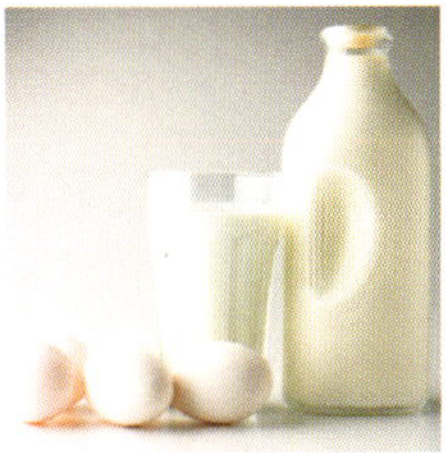

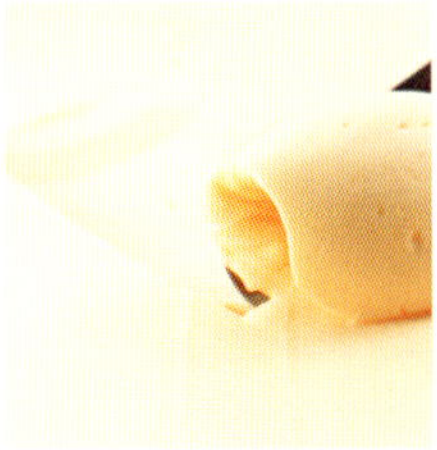

THE LONG AND SHORT OF THE MATTER

Farhan and Benny are the proverbial small and big pals. Both are 10 years old, but there's Farhan, who is small-built, and never seems to put on weight. And then there's Benny, who looks at least 16!

Both their respective mothers despair, each trying to find a balance for her child. Farhan's Mum feeds him the choicest of foods, but he remains skinny. Benny, with his voracious appetite, seems to need a new wardrobe every three months! Both need to assess and revise their eating habits and diet.

Farhan, the underweight child, could just be genetically thin, or have a very high metabolic rate. For children like Farhan, there is no need to press the panic button. The solution is to ensure an optimal food intake and attempt to boost the child's appetite. Exercise would further stimulate appetite and maintain a level of fitness. Regular meals, with favourite dishes included, are a great way to make meal-times enjoyable.

Children who tend to be overweight, as Benny is, need to focus on healthy eating and regular exercise. Junk food should be kept to a minimum and small meal portions should be encouraged.

It takes a little planning, a little patience, a little creativity and a lot of love to see that your child gets the necessary nutrients to grow healthy.

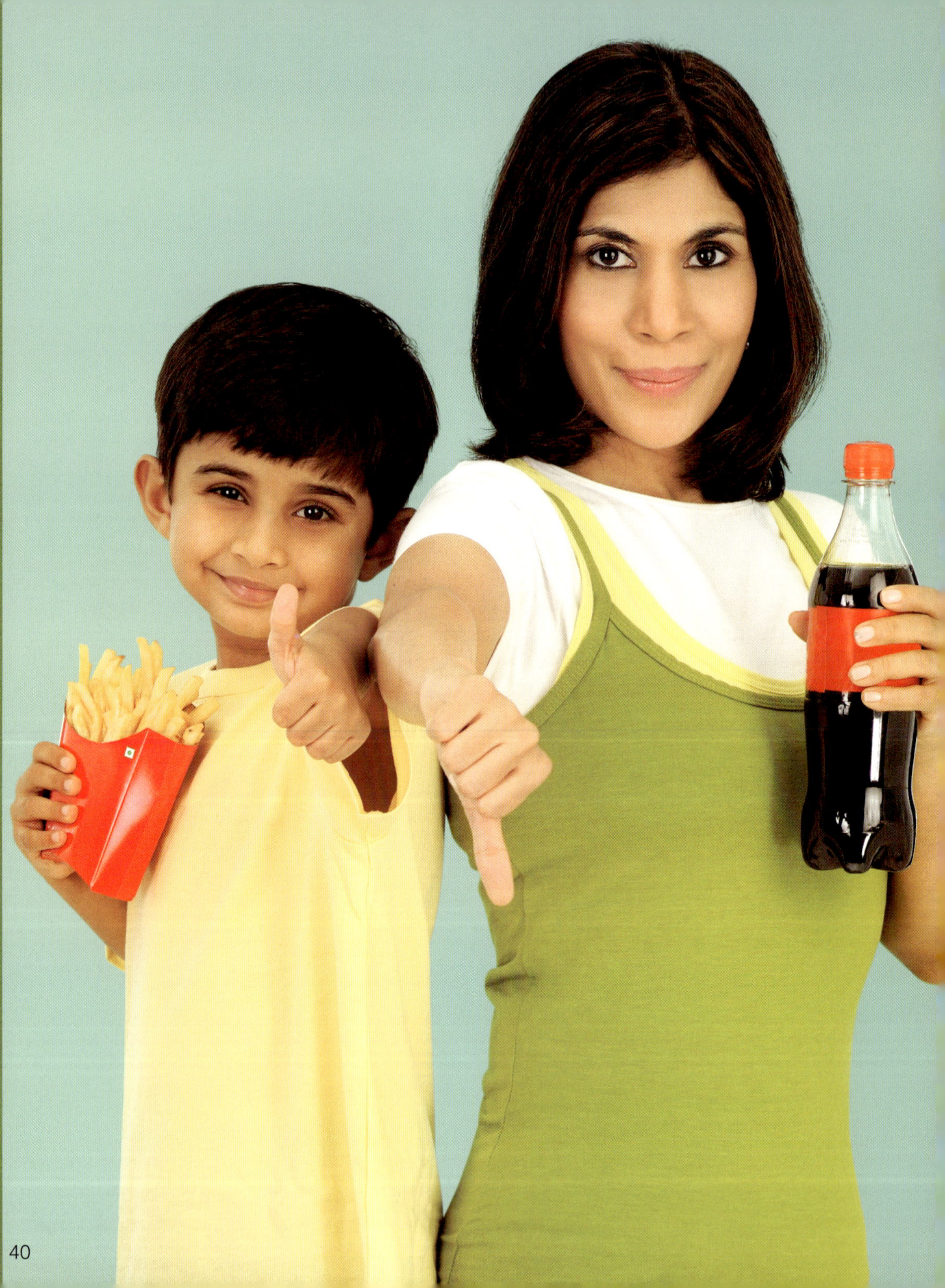

Mantra 3

Winning the great **junk food battle** is not easy. It takes **smart field strategies** to fight the craze for fast-food restaurants and to **ration junk food** consumption at home.

THE GREAT JUNK FOOD BATTLE

The "yes" and "no" arguments over junk food are a never-ending family saga. Parents try to fight the media onslaught, virtually a message-a minute, telling kids to devour chocolate bars and dig into packs of flavoured crisps. It's all about enjoying life, say the advertisers. It's all about picking up bad habits, getting dental cavities, and packing on the kilos, say parents. And the battle rages on.

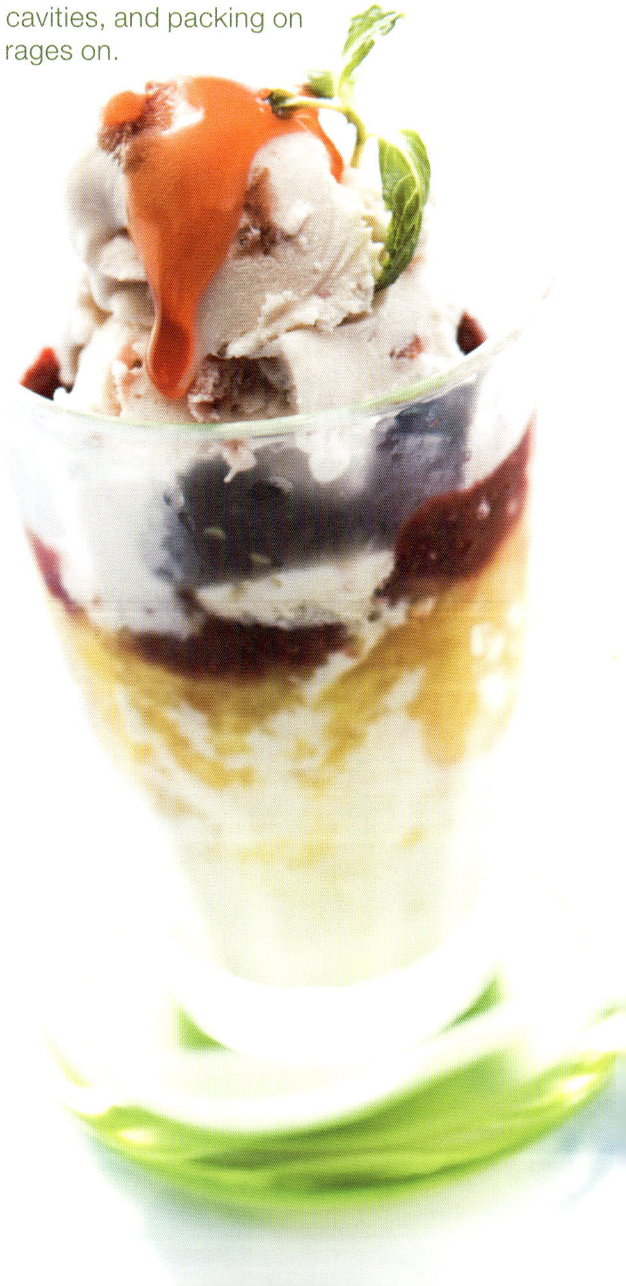

Sure, snack indulgences do have their place. Can you imagine a kid who shuns fast food restaurants and says no to candy? It ain't happening. But it's a battle you are fighting and it is up to you to plan your ground strategy. Smart maneuvers could turn the battle in your favour. The trick is to limit junk food consumption and find clever alternatives, known to you and me as camouflaged reinforcements!

It is common to see children delve happily into a bag of chips while watching television and washing it down with a bottle of cola. Fast food and junk food items are brilliantly engineered to appeal to the eyes and palate. Think junk food and you see some scary images floating before you....

- A child preoccupied with a big bag of chips, while the mother is busy shopping.
- A child watching television, mindlessly tucking into a bag of munchies.
- Kids being bribed, rewarded and cajoled with a burger or a sundae.

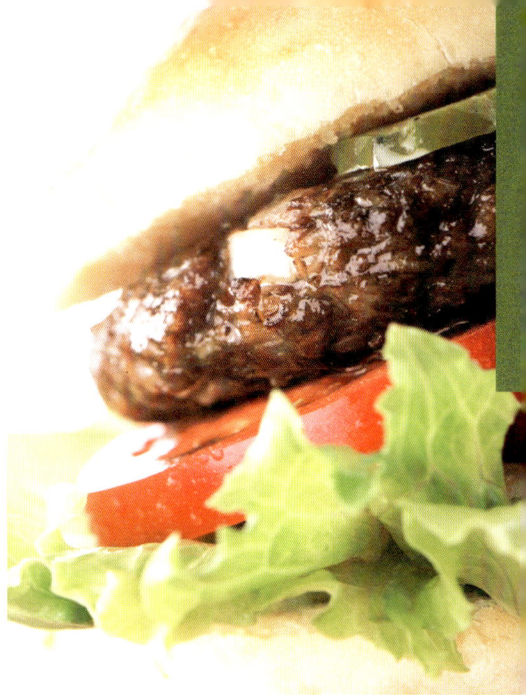

When I initially started teaching group fitness classes, some mums would have their children sitting outside the class with a packet of chips, watching their mums exercise. The mothers were happy to see the children enjoying the treat, not even aware that they were turning their kids into junk food addicts!

Allowing free and unfettered access to junk food, even using junk food as a reward, sends the wrong message to the child. With overt parental sanction, children think it's OK to eat junk as and when they please.

I have seen kids, as they get older, hanging out with friends at fast food parlours, consuming fries and ice cream as diet staples. Why does this happen? It happens because some parents genuinely don't know any better.

With the fast food trend on the rise, childhood lifestyle diseases like juvenile diabetes should come as no surprise. Parents must sit up and take notice. Before it's too late.

Let's take a minute to define junk food. Pre-packaged snack food, chocolates and packaged sweets, carbonated soft drinks, and fast food items like pizza and burgers are all examples of junk food. Manufacturers process the raw ingredients, often adding hydrogenated oils, trans-fats and monosodium glutamate, to enhance taste and prolong the shelf life of the product.

Industrially processed trans-fatty acids are typically produced from vegetable oils by a hydrogenated process that makes them solid. The solid form makes fat easier and cheaper to transport and store. Foods with a high trans-fat content have therefore been extensively promoted by the manufacturers and marketers.

A high intake of trans-fats can raise low-density cholesterol levels and increase the risk for cardiovascular disease. Trans-fats are mostly found in fast food items like French fries, cakes, hamburgers and in packaged foods such as crackers, chips, cookies and biscuits.

FACT-O-Meter

The American Heart Association recommends no more than 1 percent of calories - 1 to 3 grams per day - from trans fats.

Why is junk food and fast food so popular?

Junk food is easily available, convenient, needs little or no preparation, and is usually consumed on the go. Just what a young person is looking for! Children, especially over 12 years of age, tend to eat away from home much more than kids did 20 years ago. Fast food is often the default choice. Not only is it convenient and easy to grab, it's also tasty and cheap. And fast food joints also serve as great teenage hangout places.

But, as we well know, junk food manufacturers and fast food restaurants are not concerned with a child's health. It is not their business. Their job is to cater to the taste buds! A large burger meal with fries and a fizzy drink can contain more than half of the total daily recommendation of fat and calories.

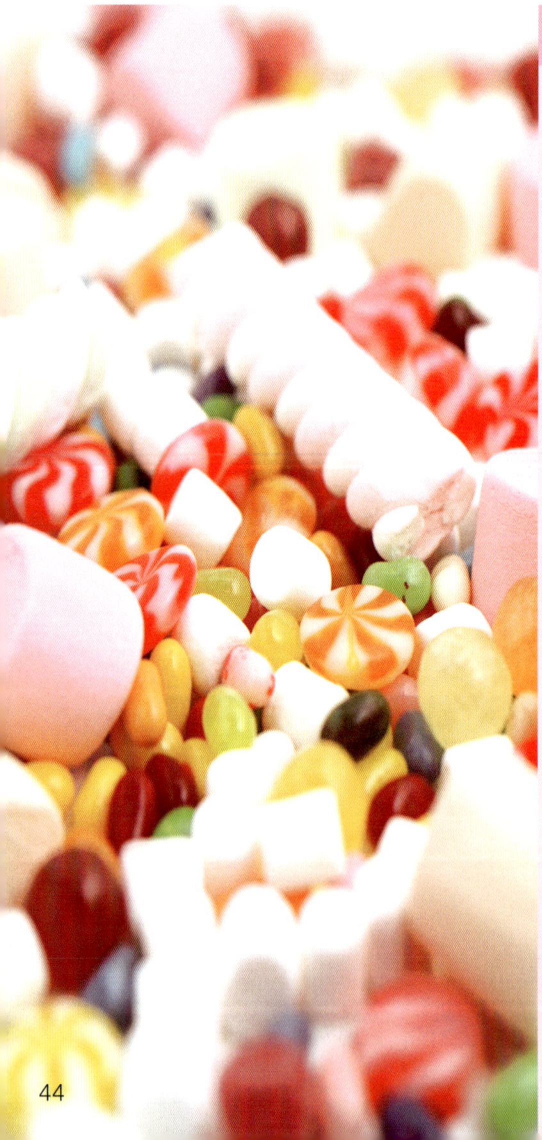

why quick-fix bribes backfire

It was difficult getting Rohan to finish his dinner without daily tantrums. So his Mom started promising ice-cream, or any sweet treat, if he finished his meal. The treat became the goal, making dinner a chore to get through with, so that he could get to his treat. This became a hard-to-break habit, creating an unhealthy eating pattern.

Let me give you another example. My friend's daughter, Manisha, hated boiled eggs. Her mother tried the "you-eat-it-I'll-treat-you" syndrome. The right option would have been to offer Manisha eggs in another form, as an omelette, or scrambled with pepper and herbs. Instead her Mom offered her a jelly sweet or chocolate animal biscuit as a reward.

Often, junk food is used as a reward, as a way to mollify the child. This is an unhealthy precedent, creating problems rather than solving them. Look at it from the kid's perspective. "Here is my Dad, offering me candy and chocolates as a reward, there must be something really special about these treats, because my parents seem to think so!"

A much better solution would be to explain to the child why he or she is being asked to eat a certain food. Every child wants to grow tall and look good. These are great incentives for your child to drink up the milk and finish the veggies. So reason things out, and see how smoothly the kids fall in line!

TIP

There will be times when your child is in a good mood, receptive and ready to learn. Use the opportunity to teach your child about the pitfalls of junk food. Explain why advertising and peer pressure are not good enough reasons to succumb.

comfort food

Parents are supposed to feed their children. That is how nature meant things to be. Mothers get tremendous emotional satisfaction watching their children eat, an experience that deepens the bond between mother and child. For you as a parent, it is one of the biggest joys of life when you see your child blooming in your care.

But sometimes, the boundaries between feeding a child and emotionally caring for the child get blurred. This is when food becomes "comfort food". Be wary of using food as bait to praise a child, punish a child, soothe feelings or express affection.

Consistently using food in this manner can build an emotional attachment to food as a comforter. Once your child starts connecting food with emotions, it becomes a complex, lifelong dependency. Food then becomes the safe haven in times of stress and strain.

- If your daughter appears bored, try to get her interested in a toy or game.
- If your son wants some of your time, take a few moments and give him your attention.
- If your child is hungry, provide a healthy snack.
- If your child needs a reward, offer a big hug instead of a sugary treat.

Catch 'em young

Sometimes, even children who have healthy eating habits may veer towards ready-to-eat, high-fat processed food as a preferred choice. Often these influences come from peers who may not have parental supervision at home.

The older children become, the more difficult it is to modify their eating habits. By about 10 to 12 years of age, as you have probably discovered, kids develop high levels of resistance and refuse to follow instructions! It is therefore best to teach and train them in the early years.

Of course, children must be able to understand what you are saying. Many child psychologists consider 4 years to be an optimum age when children understand what you are telling them and are still at an age when they listen.

Once-in-a-while

If your daughter is a lollipop lover and can't do without her daily quota, you might be tempted to put a stop to the junk food habit. But instead of forbidding the treat, it's better to allow an occasional indulgence, in controlled amounts. To make sure poor eating habits do not interfere with good nutrition, restricting junk food is vital.

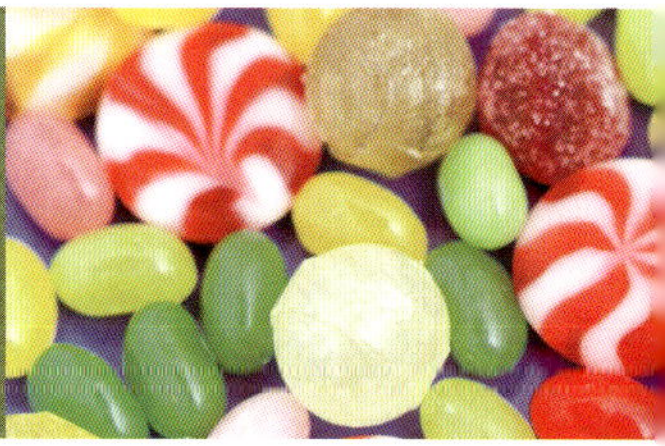

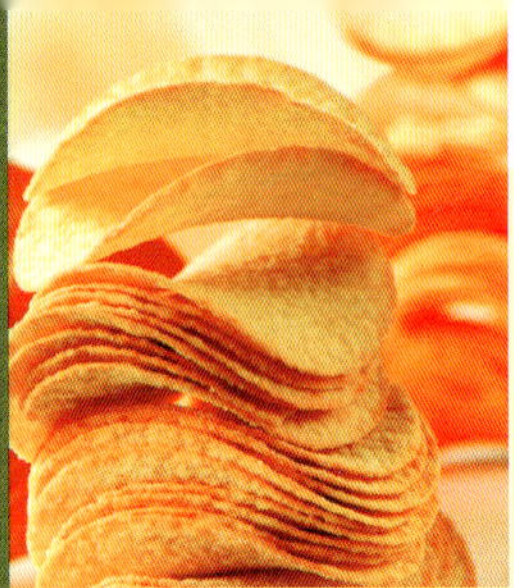

FIT guard

Battling the junk food habit is a bit like teaching children to handle money. Allow them access, then over time, let them use their judgment to make smart, sensible choices. If they demonstrate a sense of responsibility, you can give them further freedom.

In this way, children learn to eat well, indulge occasionally, and, in the long term, model an eating pattern that works for their lifestyle.

Q. Then the question arises, is junk food bad food?

A. No food is bad. But when food contributes more calories than nutrients, the problem of empty calories versus nutrition becomes something to consider. While junk food cannot be banned or excluded from a child's diet, the quantity and frequency of consumption must be controlled.

Watch out, your child is watching!

Children are quick to pick up adult attitudes about food. So beware of the signals you send out. A client of mine, Sita, had a tough time feeding her son a variety of foods during meal-times. Sita's own meals consisted of roti wraps, sometimes with veggies, or with cottage cheese. Her son couldn't understand why he was expected to eat "everything", while Mom could get away with a roti wrap.

Modifying existing eating patterns is never easy. Unhealthy food habits don't develop overnight. Getting rid of established patterns takes time and patience. It helps to remember you are your child's best role model. If you make healthy living your priority – what you eat, when you eat, how much you eat, and how often you exercise – you are setting an example for your child to follow.

How to camouflage junk food

Call it your hidden field strategy! If your child is crazy about crisps, buy a small quantity occasionally. But mix the crisps up with a healthier ingredient, such as kurmura, popcorn, or chana, and you are upping the nutrition quotient of the snack. If your child loves sugary, flavoured breakfast cereal, add a small amount of high fibre wheat flakes or muesli to the sugared cereal. If your child craves carbonated fizzy drinks, dilute the extra sweet drink with a measure of natural unsweetened fruit juice.

Mohan loved fizzy lemon drinks. His Mum would mix nimbu pani with the flavoured drink in a 50- 50 proportion. Once Mohan got used to this, his Mom added a ¾ proportion of nimbu pani. Mohun was happy - he couldn't tell the difference and his Mom was equally happy - because she could!

Kid friendly kitchen

One of my clients, Rajul, made life really simple. She dedicated a couple of shelves in her kitchen cabinet to accommodate her kids' snacks. So when the children say, "I'm hungry", or when their little friends come over home, she heads straight for her kiddy snack shelves!

FACT-O-Meter

The fact is kids eat too much fat, so find ways to restrict your child's intake at around 30-35 percent of total calories consumed in a day.

Art of substitution

If you can get away with total substitution, nothing like it. You may need to alternate the junk food and the healthy options for an initial period, then gradually phase out the junk altogether.

Offer alternatives that do not compromise on taste, but are high on nutrition. Remember, a little bit of hype around the forthcoming treat never hurts. After all, if your children can be sold on a food product, thanks to some clever advertising, you too can use the same communication skills to get your kids hooked onto home-made goodies!

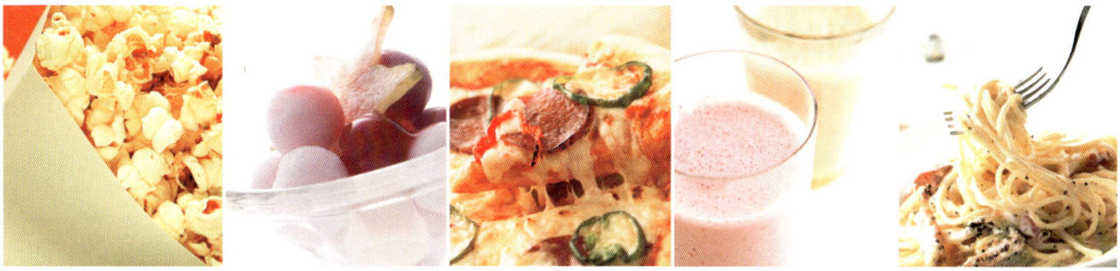

Here are some options to try:

- POPCORN instead of a packet of chips
- FROZEN FRUIT JUICE ICE LOLLIES instead of ice-cream
- WHOLE WHEAT BASE PIZZA instead of regular pizza
- VEGGIE CUTLET MULTIGRAIN BURGER instead of a regular burger
- FRUIT SMOOTHIE instead of milkshakes
- ROTI ROLL WITH SPICY CHICKEN/PANEER FILLING instead of a Frankie
- STRAWBERRY/BANANA DIPPED IN FRUIT YOGHURT instead of dessert
- HOME-MADE NIMBU PANI instead of fizzy drinks
- WHOLE WHEAT PASTA & VEGGIES IN CREAMY SAUCE instead of regular pasta in creamy sauce
- GRILLED/BAKED CHICKEN NUGGETS instead of deep fried chicken

Read the label

Given the range of convenience foods available, consumers need to carefully consider what each one has to offer. It is worth taking the time to look at the labels, before making a decision whether to buy it or not.

Restrict convenience foods that are high in sugar and fat, particularly trans-fats. A quick scan of the ingredients can be very useful. Trans-fats are mostly found in fast foods like burgers and fries, and in packaged foods such as crisps, cookies and biscuits.

The good news is that, today, there are many healthy savoury snack foods on store shelves. Khakra, low fat bhel puri, soya nuggets, baked chakli, and multigrain biscuits make tasty choices. With consumers becoming more health conscious, new products keep entering the market, so keep a lookout for what's in store.

Q. Should children eat a low-fat diet?

A. No. Restrictive diets are not recommended for children. Despite the bad press, fat is not the enemy. For young children in particular, fat and cholesterol play an important part in brain development. It is important that children eat a varied diet with 30-35 percent of calories from fat.

Do's and don'ts for healthy eating

- Do keep ready-to-eat healthy snacks accessible when your child gets hungry.
- Do provide structured eating and snacking times each day.
- Do encourage small, "try it" portions of a tablespoon or two.
- Do put your work away and concentrate on your meal.
- Do help your child cultivate an adventurous approach to different foods and textures.
- Do restrict pocket money spent on junk food.
- Do eat together as a family and offer nutritious choices.
- Do encourage your child to sit down and eat slowly.
- Don't use dessert as an incentive or a way to beat boredom or stress.
- Don't eat in front of the television.
- Don't encourage the habit of eating at fast food joints.
- Don't eat on the move, or while rushing off somewhere.

weight watch

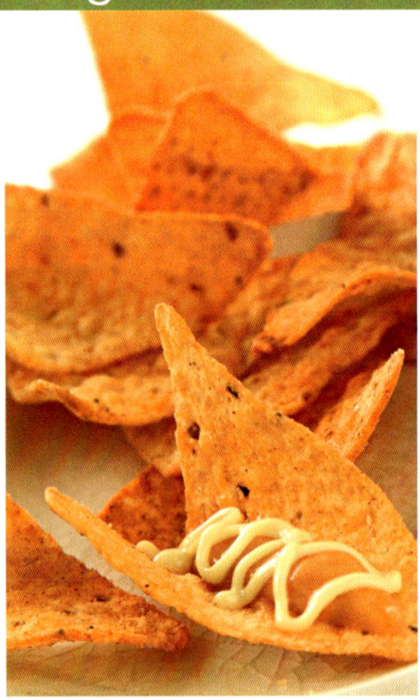

An increasing number of children are overweight, and, if there is no intervention, approximately 80 percent of these children are likely to become overweight adults.

Shyam, a 12-year old, loved eating his bag of chips during tuck time in school. He also treated himself to at least three pizzas a week, and a couple of burgers. He was given pocket money so that he could pick up food after school and after swimming.

"Childhood is the age to indulge, children should be given special treats", said his Mum, who expressed her affection towards Shyam by allowing him frequent indulgences. "This is his age to enjoy food, his childhood fat will melt away as he grows," she believed.

But as Shyam grew older, his mother regretted encouraging the junk habit, because, by that time, her son refused to eat healthier foods, despite his expanding waistline.

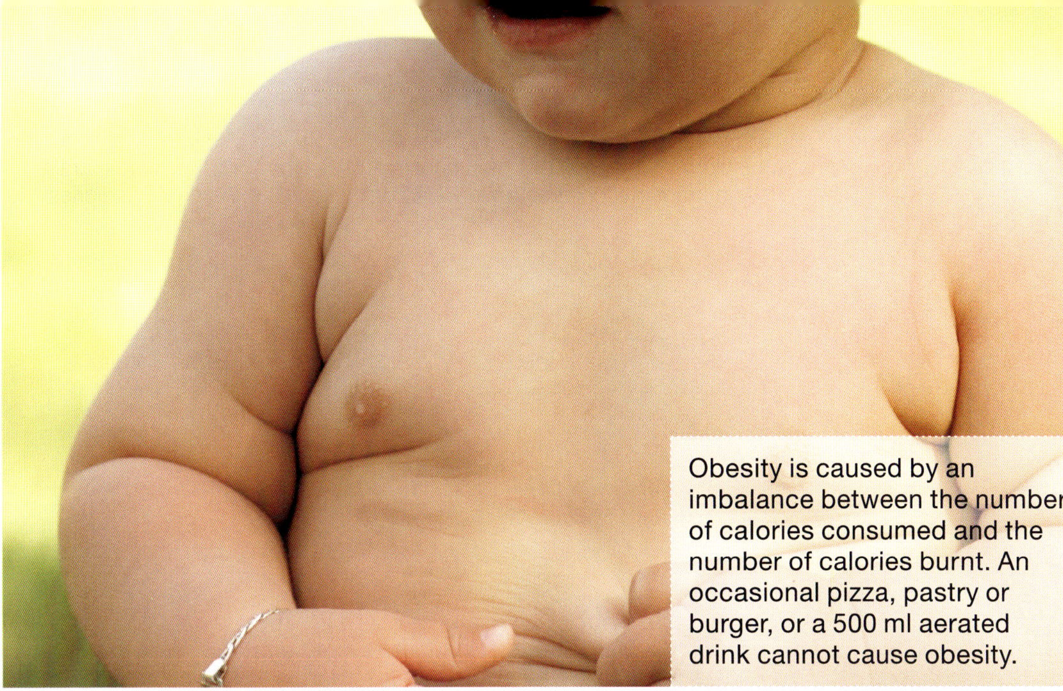

Obesity is caused by an imbalance between the number of calories consumed and the number of calories burnt. An occasional pizza, pastry or burger, or a 500 ml aerated drink cannot cause obesity.

Some obesity-causing factors to avoid

- Easy access to food establishments
- Unhealthy eating patterns
- Eating tied to leisure
- Larger portion sizes
- Cravings for fast food and eating triggers
- Inactivity
- Family outings and interests revolving around food

FACT-O-Meter

Despite the popular belief that obesity in childhood is a benign condition, children do not outgrow their puppy fat. It is statistically proven that the longer a child has been overweight, the greater the chances of that child being overweight during adolescence and adulthood.

The consequences of obesity are not just health-related, but can shatter a child's confidence. To illustrate the point, I will use my student Shamim as an example.

Shamim, a beautiful 13-year old, hated going out. Being overweight, she shied away from family gatherings, found excuses not to socialize with her friends, and was always unhappy with what she wore. She lived in a joint family. Her aunt, who was plump too, realized what the matter was, and boosted Shamim's spirits by taking her shopping, asking her to highlight her beautiful eyes, to smile and stay happy. She also coaxed Shamim to join a gym. (That's when Shamim came to me.)

Children who have weight problems are sensitive about it. It is best not to focus too closely on the weight issue and certainly not to make a joke of it, as some younger family members might do. It is far more productive to initiate a healthy eating and exercise plan and to help your child through it. Try not to criticize your child's efforts. Provide plenty of comfort, attention and encouragement and watch your child respond.

home sweet home

Parents exert a huge influence on their children's environment. At a subconscious level, family members influence each other in key lifestyle choices, such as healthy eating and leisure activities. Chances are, if parents are obese, children could have a tendency to be obese too.

By making positive choices like nutrient-rich foods, regular meals at the family dining table and time together for physical activity, parents are setting an example for children to follow. All of these factors could play a crucial role in preventing obesity.

If certain lifestyle patterns need to be modified, it has to be a collective family effort. A single family member, in isolation, cannot work towards weight loss. Team effort wins the day!

FIT Alert

Parents who exert too much control over their child's food intake, or promote a highly restrictive diet, may cause children to overeat when the opportunity is available.

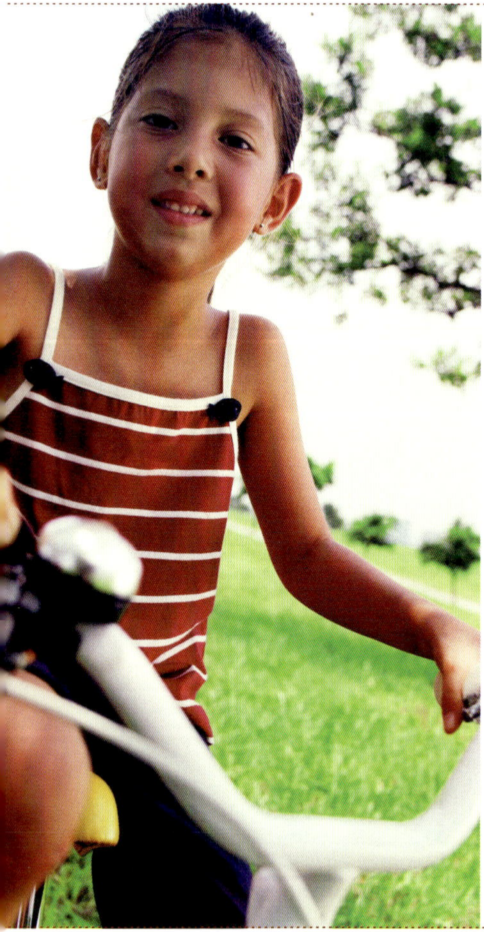

Take charge now!

- Stock your kitchen with healthy food like fruits, vegetables, whole grain foods and unsaturated fat.
- Reduce the frequency of outings to fast-food outlets and restaurants.
- Try new recipes and tweak family favourites with healthier ingredients. Kids enjoy healthy home-made versions of their favourite junk food.
- Make lighter food choices when possible. Replace cream in puddings with evaporated skimmed milk. Eat egg white instead of the whole egg. Whole grain instead of refined products. Low-fat instead of full fat.
- Build physical activity into the daily routine. Let your children participate in household chores like washing the car, walking the dog. Go on regular family outings, that involve physical activity, for instance, weekend cycling.
- Explain to your kids why healthy eating is essential. Don't talk down to them, don't reprimand. Give them information, answer their queries, take them to a library, access the internet for information. Tell them that junk food is OK once in a while, but cannot become the staple diet.
- Praise your kids' efforts. This support goes a long way when they are under peer pressure and need the confidence to stick to their new goals. Give them responsibility. Encourage children to plan, shop and occasionally, to cook with you. Consult them about food choices and they feel more involved.

Q: What do you do if your child needs to lose weight?

A: To lose weight you need to create a calorie deficit. A weight loss of 1 pound, that is roughly ½ a kilo per week, is safe. To lose 1 pound a week you need to cut back on 500 calories a day. That is a total of 3500 calories a week. The best way to achieve this is by reducing your child's calorie intake and increasing calorie expenditure through exercise.

Q: Should you count calories when planning meals for your child?

A: No. You can't base a diet or food plan solely on calorie counting. The danger in this is that you might not end up following a "well-balanced" eating plan. Growing children need nutrients from various food groups such as proteins, carbohydrates, fats, vitamins and minerals. Even skipping meals is not healthy, as it leads to irregular eating habits and slows down the body's metabolism.

Consult a dietician

Children need a nutritionally balanced diet. Placing diet restrictions on a child could lead to nutritional deficiencies, which could compromise long term health and growth. For this reason, it is essential to get advice from your physician or from a qualified dietician.

GET FIT TACTICS

Shop	Shop from a list. Pre-plan your child's requirements so you get what you need.
Plan	Plan healthy menus that your child will enjoy. Encourage eating meals at scheduled times. Store junk food out of sight.
Encourage	Do not encourage the habit of lingering at the table. Encourage your child to leave the table after eating meals, to avoid overeating.
Move on	Don't get discouraged by an occasional setback.
Avoid entertainment eating	Avoid watching television while eating. It only leads to mindless eating habits.
Reward	Praise or rewards like a t-shirt, book, a picnic or a movie work wonders.
Educate	Substitute high fat foods with low-fat options. Learn nutritional values of food, experiment with low fat recipes.
Get physical	Find an activity that your child enjoys. Encourage regular exercise.
Can do approach	Avoid words like "never" or "always". Counter negative thoughts with positive ones. A setback is okay, but getting back is what is important.

When you do take the kids out for an occasional fast food treat, some of the guidelines here will help you to make the right choices.

- Never order "super size" items just because it's a cheaper deal.
- Avoid two-for-the-price-of-one offers because your children will just end up over-eating.
- Say no to extras such as bacon and more cheese
- Try a mixed salad on the side, corn on the cob or some fruit.

1 pound = 3500 calories

If your child eliminates the 250-calorie chocolate bar and burns 250-calories by running 3 miles, he would create a calorie deficit of 500 calories. Do this every day and he will create a deficit of 3500 calories in one week.

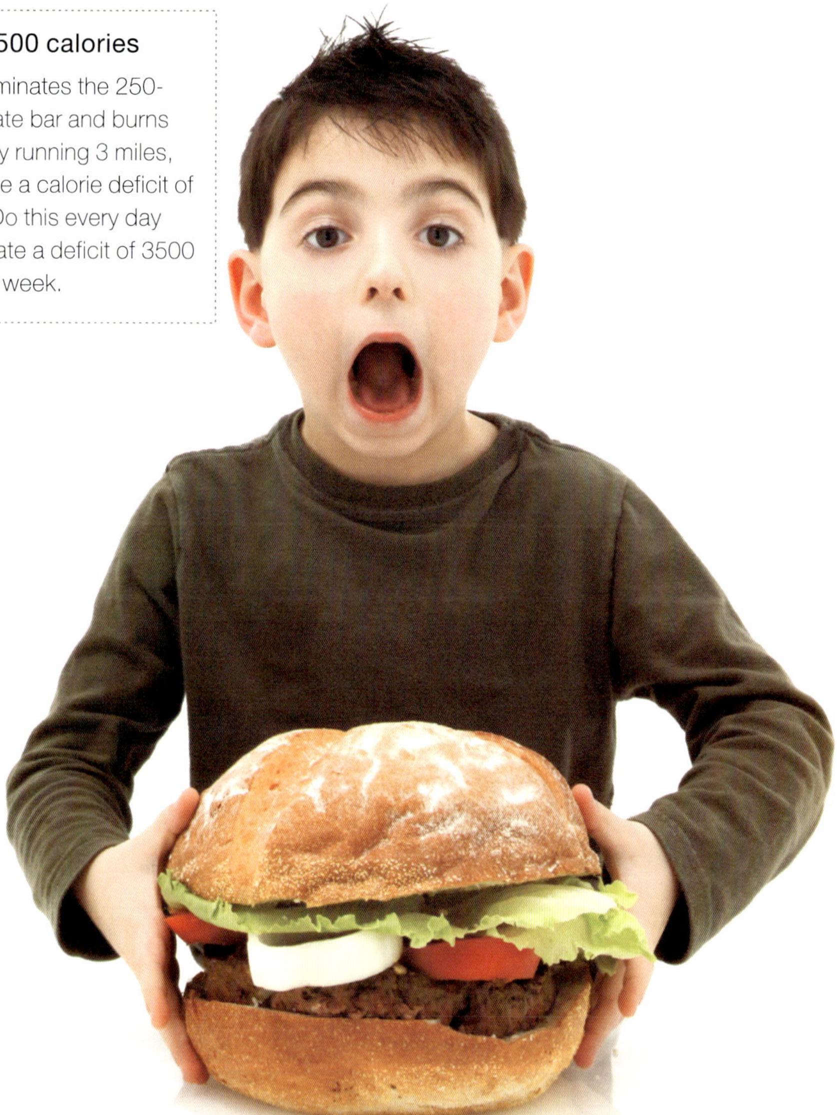

FIT Tips

1 Start small

Small changes are the easiest to make. Your child can try switching from milkshakes to low fat badam milk or skimmed milk lassi.

Another practical option is to cut down on the quantity of junk food, rather than give it up altogether. Even small changes such as these work in the long run.

2 Ration, but don't rule out

As children grow older and have money to spend, they tend to consume more snacks from stores or fast-food restaurants. Parents need to set limits, but also be realistic. Both sides can learn to compromise a little bit, so that arguments over food don't become a full blown war!

3 De-code the signals

Aromas, association of some delightful culinary experience, television commercials, are all powerful stimuli that make your child's mouth water! Everyone has their own buttons which, when pressed, trigger "I want food" signals. Observe what creates these food triggers in your child. Is it habit, boredom, depression or is it just knowing that there is yummy food in the house?

Sometimes, when your child is alone at home, food becomes a magnet. Then he or she will succumb to temptation, often indulging, even over-indulging, in all the junk food they can find. Of course, this makes them feel guilty. To avoid the eat-everything-you-can-lay your-hands-on trap, teach your child the Count Ten Trick or the Drink Water Distraction! Biting into an apple or crunching up a cucumber slice are also great ways to overcome the bingeing urge.

4 One victory at a time

If your child is not amenable to re-vamping his or her diet, introduce the change very gradually. Remember, treating obesity doesn't happen overnight. Wean your child away from bad habits slowly and steadily. Making lifestyle changes can be stressful, but some effort and planning, and most important, a positive attitude, will certainly win the battle.

FACT-O-Meter

Skimmed milk gets 5 % of its calories from fat while the fat in whole milk constitutes 51% of its total calorific value.

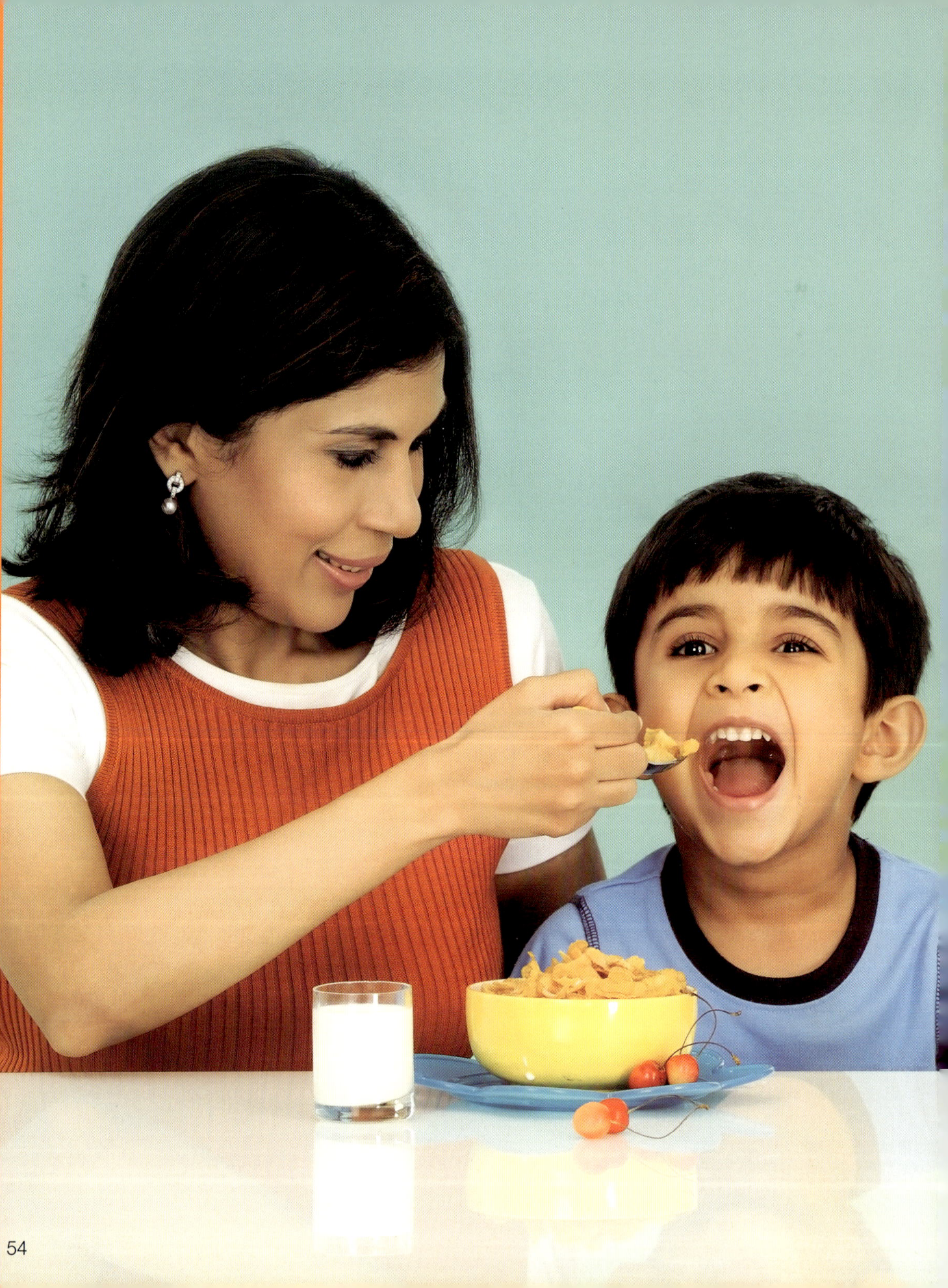

Mantra 4

Breakfast is a make-or-break morning starter. Children who enjoy a **hearty breakfast** before school are more **mentally alert** and **energetic,** while breakfast-skippers tend to perform under par.

WAKE UP TO BREAKFAST

Good morning, parents. It's time for breakfast, the most challenging meal of the day. I know it's hard. As the clock ticks, you are trying to find school socks and toast bread at the same time. You are busy fixing your child's hair just as the milk starts to boil over. To top it all, the lunch box is waiting to be packed. If this sounds like a typical morning, take a deep breath. And relax. With a little bit of planning, breakfast can be smooth and hassle-free. And your child can enjoy a hearty, healthy breakfast before heading off to school.

It is extremely important to make sure your child does not miss out on breakfast. This is because breakfast is the first meal of the day, after a long gap of 10 to 12 hours.

A satisfying breakfast helps your child to be active and energetic through the morning. If breakfast is not adequate, there is a dip in glucose levels in the body. Your child will be lethargic and listless, with a short attention span in school. Research shows that children who eat a good breakfast focus better in school as compared to children who don't eat a hearty breakfast in the mornings. The brain needs food to function, just as the body does!

Even more disturbing, children who are deprived at breakfast-time may have nutritional deficiencies. Insufficient calcium and protein intakes lead to poor muscle growth and bone development. Breakfast-skippers are also more likely to face the problem of obesity. This is because your child will feel more hungry as the day progresses and end up eating more in the latter part of the day.

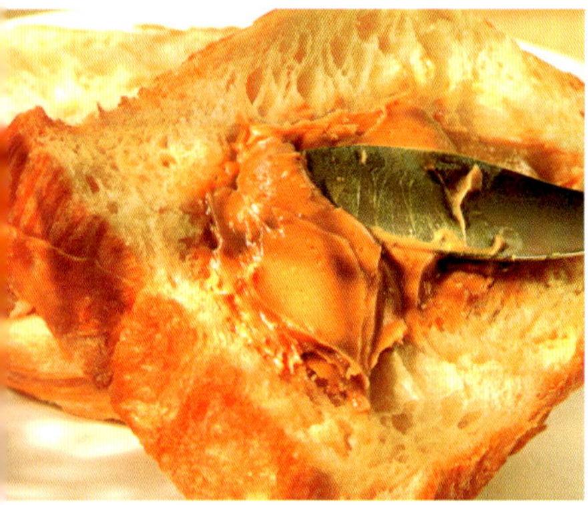

Q. With so much at stake, how do you make sure your child does not leave home on an empty stomach?

A. Anuj, my cousin's son, was always behind schedule for school. This meant he had no time for breakfast. I remember his mother running after him with a bowl of cereal in her hand, feeding him, as Anuj packed his school bag and put on his uniform. He barely managed a few spoons before he ran off to catch his bus. His Mom was left standing helplessly, the unfinished breakfast still in her hands. By this point, she was so fed up, that Anuj's Mom sought my help in rectifying the situation. I suggested she change her approach.

First of all, she had to ensure Anuj had packed his school bag and kept his uniform ready the night before. This automatically gave him more time in the morning. Then, she made it a point to serve up his favourite foods for breakfast. Anuj loved peanuts. He adored bananas. So she started giving him peanut butter on toast. Or sago (sabudana) khichadi, with roasted peanuts.

Bananas were an equally versatile option. She made banana milkshakes, put sliced bananas in custard (made the night before), or, if he was really late, just gave him a couple of bananas to eat on his way to school!

Like Anuj's Mom, you too can make adjustments to suit your child. If your kid likes eggs, keep eggs boiled and ready from the night before. Or whip up a wholesome vegetable omelette.

Some children are very happy with honey or chocolate added to milk, to break the monotony of drinking milk every day. To avoid getting your child hooked on chocolate, you could just sprinkle some chocolate powder over smoothies or plain milk.

fibre is filling

Nothing like a filling, fibre-rich breakfast to jump start your child's day. A high-fibre breakfast goes a long way in sustaining your child all the way till the mid morning break in school.

Breakfast offers lots of fibre-rich choices. Your child can consume whole-grain toast, fresh fruit or cereals like oats or muesli. To give your child the maximum advantage from fibre, here's what you can do -

- Offer whole fruits rather than juice. Most of the fibre in fruit is found in skin, seeds and pulp.
- Use a variety of cereals - bran, oatmeal. whole-wheat flour, muesli, cornflakes, ragi, jawar, brown rice and barley.
- Add vegetables to dishes like poha or upma. Over-cooking reduces the fibre content of vegetables, so steam or cook the veggies only until tender, but firm to bite.
- Add nuts, seeds, sprouts in your child's cereal.

FIBRE CONTENT OF SOME FOODS

FOOD GROUP	QUANTITY	GRAMS OF FIBRE
Beans and lentils		
Lentils cooked	½ cup	7.8
Kidney beans cooked	½ cup	7.3
Chickpeas cooked	½ cup	5.3
Cereals		
Oatmeal cooked	1 cup	4
Raisin bran	¾ cup	5
Bran flakes	¾ cup	5
Breads and grains		
Brown rice cooked	½ cup	2
Whole-wheat bread	1 slice	2
Fruits		
Pear with skin	1	4
Apple with skin	1	3.7
Peach with skin	1	3.4
Figs dried	2	4

WHEN YOU ARE PRESSED FOR TIME

We all know breakfast is important but often, as a working parent, you could be pressed for time. My mother always told me, over and over again, to have a good breakfast before I stepped out. She herself took good care to eat a balanced, nutritious breakfast, and, as a kid, I took the cue from her. Nowadays, the ground reality is a little different! Many kids see their working parents rushing through breakfast, or skipping breakfast altogether. They do not, therefore, feel it is as important as Mom is making it out to be.

Q. As a parent, what can you do to help your kid start right?

A. If you do not eat a proper breakfast yourself, now's the time to start! Because your child will pick up the breakfast habit from you and follow your lead. Yes, it means preparing a wholesome breakfast, sitting down at the dining table, and consuming it in an unhurried manner. With your hectic morning schedule, this may not be easy. But for the health for your family, it is essential.

Breakfast does not have to be an elaborate affair. Keep it as simple, as basic as possible. Plan and prepare in advance, preferably the previous night. If you plan a vegetable upma, for example, keep the semolina (rawa) cleaned and roasted, ready to cook. Have some diced vegetables ready-frozen, so you can just sauté them in oil and get started. Grind the chutney and store in a container in the fridge.

If your family prefers toast, use bread options like whole wheat, multigrain, rye, even breads with seeds, nuts and dry fruit. Make sure the butter is out of the fridge, so it's not frozen solid! Imaginative toppings on toast will work wonders - honey, home made fruit jams or chutneys, cottage cheese, kidney beans (rajma) in tomato sauce, peanut butter, scrambled eggs, a mayonnaise or yoghurt spread with chopped vegetables – be creative.

I am a big fan of cereal, so if your child likes cornflakes, or, on a cold day, would like to eat some porridge, your breakfast problem is solved. Every day, you could add different fruits to the bowl of cereal, to make it fun.

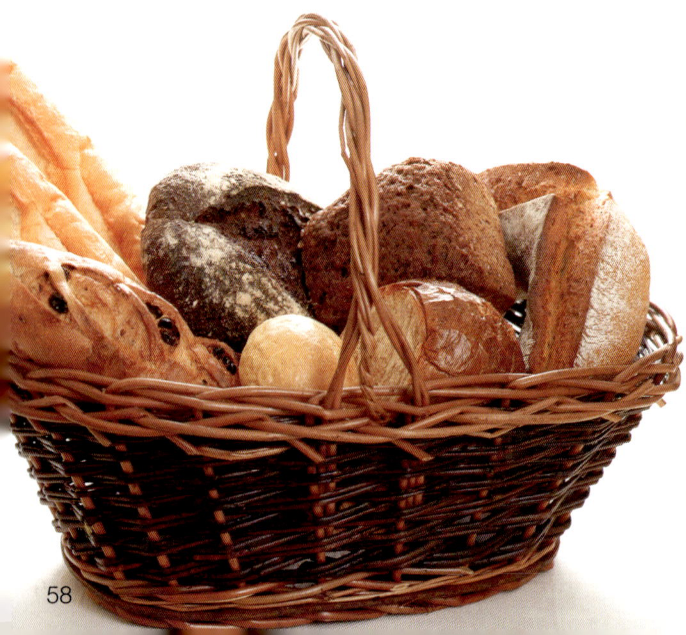

FACT-O-Meter

When your child consumes a good breakfast, the body stores glucose in the liver as glycogen. The liver releases this glucose as bursts of energy throughout the day. If your child skips breakfast, the body's energy will dissipate in no time, because glycogen is in short supply.

1. Do not serve sugary breakfast cereals and donuts in the morning.
2. Buy a variety of whole-grain cereals that are low in sugar.
3. Sprinkle wheat bran or powdered flax seed (alsi) on cereal for extra fibre.
4. Make cottage cheese sandwiches, scrambled egg burritos, chicken roll-ups and other finger foods that kids can eat quickly.
5. Try to get your kids to eat breakfast sitting down instead of on the go.

Q. Are you a working Mom?

A. Supermoms need all the help they can get! If you are a working mother, planning the morning is all-important. Prepare breakfast ingredients in advance, lay the table the night before. A bowl of breakfast cereal is the easiest thing to serve, but can become boring on a daily basis.

I have listed out a few interesting breakfast options, both hot and cold, for Moms-On-The Go. With an eye on the clock, you will get a fair idea of how much time to keep aside for each breakfast item.

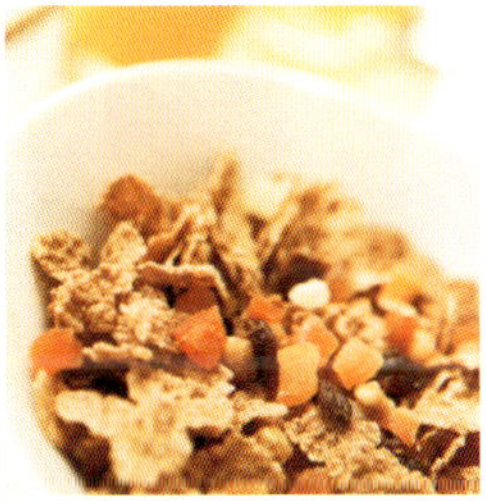

1-2 minutes

Muesli in milk

Whole-wheat toast with cottage cheese

Whipped banana yoghurt smoothie

Fruit flavoured milk

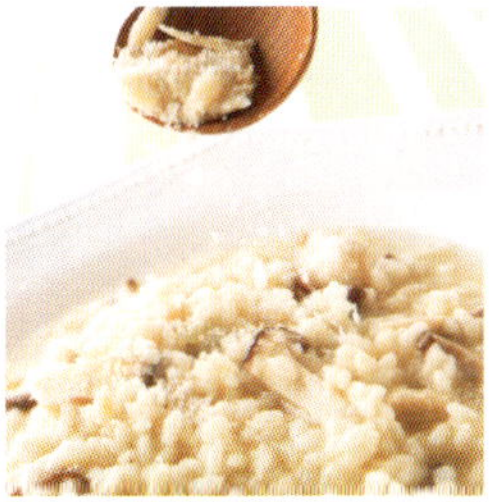

3-5 minutes

Instant oatmeal

Tinned baked beans on toast

Scrambled egg on toast

Yoghurt with assorted diced fresh fruit

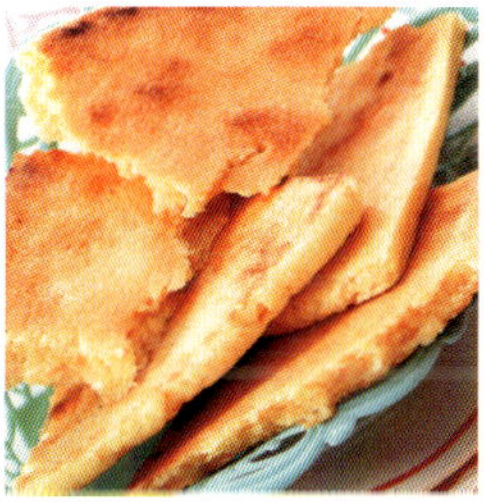

5-15 minutes

Stuffed paratha (filling can be made previous night)

Idlis (batter and chutney made previous night)

Vegetable upma

Dahlia porridge

Peas poha (boil potatoes night before, use frozen peas)

Vegetable & cheese omelette

Dosa / utthapam

I don't think you want to spend anything over 15 minutes in the kitchen! Keep experimenting with new ideas and you can serve up the most amazing breakfast in a jiffy.

FAST FORWARD

Sometimes, if your child is a slow eater, or has woken up late, you may need an emergency breakfast on hand.

- FRUIT MILKSHAKE Not only is this an instant option, your child can gulp it down in no time. Keep changing the fruit in the milk, so that your kid does get fed up! Fruits like chickoos, bananas, strawberries, apple, custard apple, or even dates, are very popular with kids.
- DRY FRUITS & NUTS Drop a large handful of almonds, cashews, raisins, figs and peanuts into a zip-lock pouch. Hand it over to your kid.
- CHEESE SANDWICH If there is no time to toast bread, it does not matter. Simply butter the bread, fill in ready-sliced cheese and hey, an instant on-the-run sandwich is ready.
- 200ml MILK/ SOY MILK TETRA PACKS All set with their own straw, the portable tetra packs are a great on-the-go option. I would not recommend the tetra packs on a daily basis, because of the high sugar content, it is fine as an occasional "fast forward" breakfast idea.
- WHOLE FRUIT AND FRUIT JUICES An easy-to-eat fruit like an apple, pear, or banana is ideal. Just wash it well and let your child enjoy it on the way to school.

EXPERIMENT WITH DIFFERENT JUICES

- ½ cup orange juice + ½ cup apple juice
- ½ cup sweetlime juice + ½ cup pineapple juice + ½ banana puree (optional)
- ½ cup apple juice + ½ cup pineapple juice
- watermelon juice + orange juice

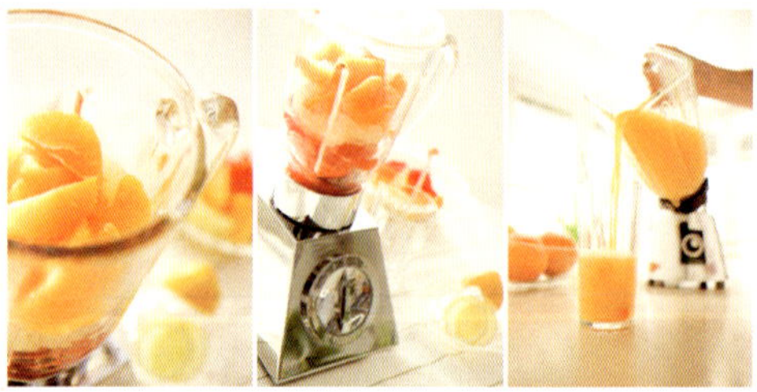

TIP: Purchasing cereal with dry fruits and nuts is expensive. Instead, buy the dry fruits and nuts separately, combine walnuts, almonds, cashews, raisins, apricots, dates, and store it in a glass container. Simply pop a handful of this into the cereal every morning.

what makes a square breakfast?

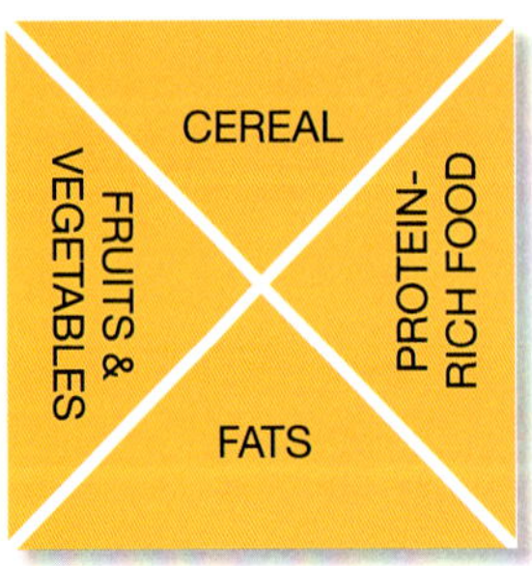

It is vital to consume a balanced breakfast with the 4 essential food groups on the table. This gives your children a head start for the day.

Cereals, fruits and vegetables, protein-rich foods and fats are the 4 essential food groups for a healthy diet. The 4 food groups ensure a balanced, wholesome breakfast.

1. **CEREALS**

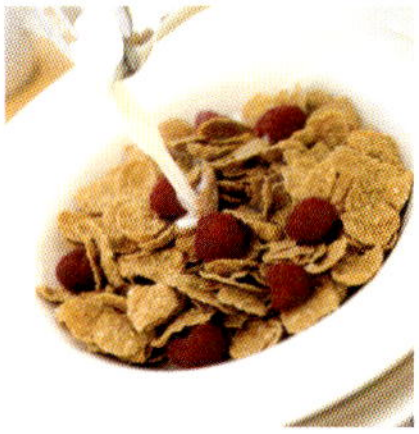

This food group makes up the bulk of your child's breakfast requirement. Cereals contain carbohydrates, a source of energy for the body and the brain. Consuming cereals in an unrefined form, such as whole-wheat bread instead of white bread, retains the valuable fibre and nutrients in the diet.

Grains like rice, wheat, barley, bajra, millet, jowar, oats, fall in this category. Also included are grain variants, including dishes like poha, sooji, upma, noodles, idlis and dosas.

2. **FRUITS or VEGETABLES**

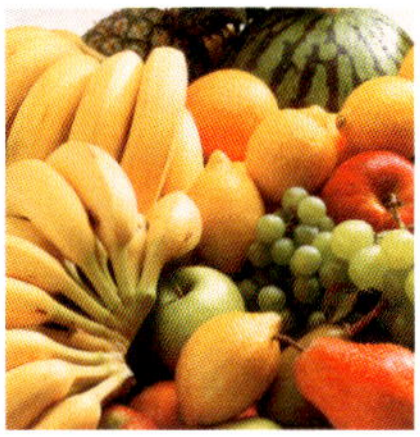

For your child's vitamin and mineral requirements, this food group is vital. The different colours in fruits and vegetables have different nutritional properties, so varying the options gives your child the full benefit of a broad range of vitamins and minerals.

Overcooking destroys natural nutrients, it is therefore important to serve vegetables in a lightly cooked form.

Locally grown seasonal fruits and vegetables give your child the benefit of nature at its best. Citrus fruits such as oranges, sweetlimes and watermelon are a light and delicious option in the summer months. Fruits such as bananas, mangoes, chikoos, sitaphal are more filling. Even dried fruits, like prunes, figs, raisins, apricots make a healthy sweet treat.

3. **PROTEIN RICH FOODS**

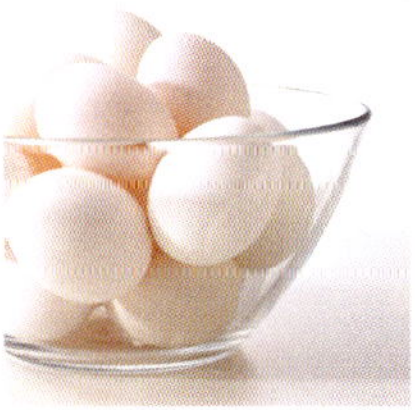

Proteins are the building blocks of your child's growth. Kids must get the protein equivalent in grams, of their weight in kilograms. For instance, if your daughter weighs 40 kilos, she should consume 40 grams of protein every day.

Non-vegetarians can derive their protein from chicken, fish, meats and eggs. Vegetarians have milk and milk products, pulses, sprouts, nuts, seeds and soya products to choose from.

4. **FATS**

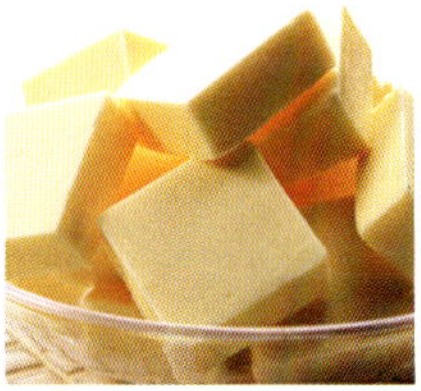

As a food group, fats should be consumed in very small quantities. However, fats are required by the body for the absorption of fat-soluble vitamins A, D, E and K.

You can choose from a variety of fats such as pure ghee, butter, olive oil and unrefined cooking oils.

For more information log on to liveactive.com

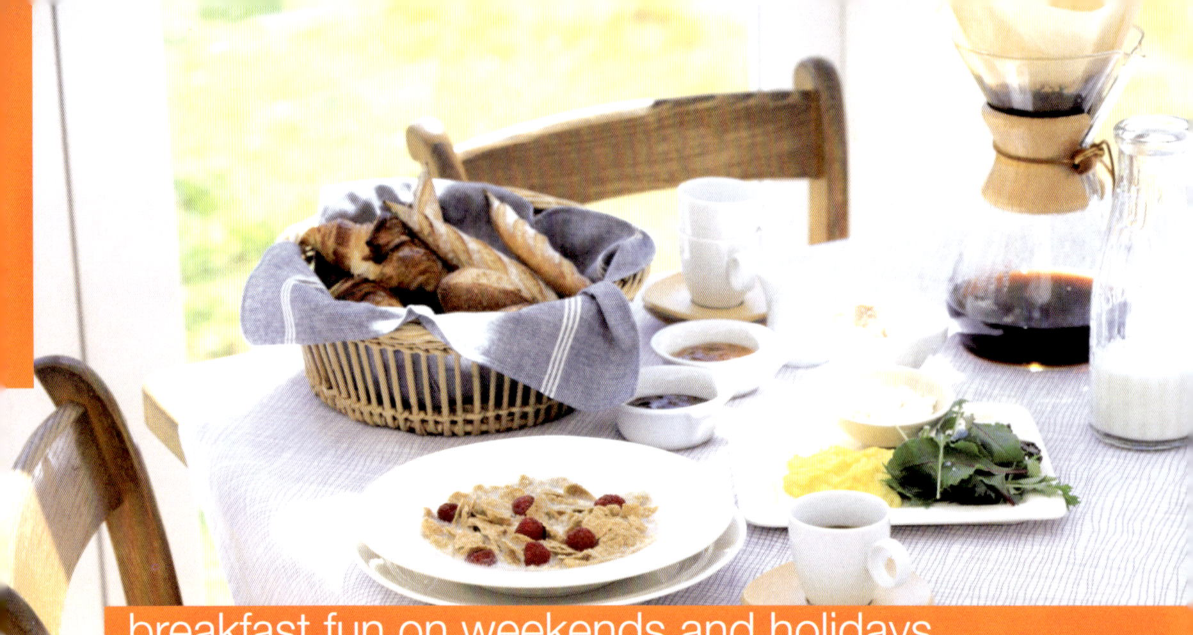

breakfast fun on weekends and holidays

A lazy morning is perfect for family bonding over breakfast. On weekends and holidays, children enjoy helping out in the kitchen. They are fascinated with the colourful array of fruits and vegetables, the fragrance of baking, and love nothing more than kneading a mountain of dough, preferably with both hands!

Make the most of it. Get them involved in a baking session or, if they are late risers, enlist their help in organizing a brunch. Make it a family event where everyone has a blast.

I have some recipes here that are sure to be a hit with the kids. And Moms, you have nothing to worry about, because these mouth-watering selections are not just breakfast treats, but amazingly healthy recipes that the whole family will enjoy.

1 banana, date and honey smoothie

Smoothies are an instant, on-the-go "meal" and I have given some all-time favourites that will go down well with your kids.

Nutrients	:	vitamins A, B1, B12, C, D, K, folic acid, calcium, iron, potassium, zinc
Preparation time	:	5 minutes
Serves	:	1
Ingredients	:	2 bananas
		2 dates
		1 teaspoon honey
		¾ cup milk
Directions	:	Buzz all the ingredients in a blender until smooth and frothy. Drink immediately.

2 chicken delight

Chicken and cheese is a classic combo, always a hot favourite with kids. The vegetables give it an extra bite, and of course, extra nutrients as well.

Nutrients : protein, vitamin A, K, D, B 12, riboflavin, niacin, calcium

Preparation time : 45 minutes

Serves : 4

Ingredients :

4 chicken breast halves

½ teaspoon seasoned salt

1 teaspoon Italian seasoning

8 to 10 French beans, in julienne strips

1 small carrot, in julienne strips or
1 cup shredded carrots

1 red pepper, in julienne strips

½ cup shredded mozzarella cheese

1 cup bottled barbecue sauce

Directions :

Preheat oven to 250 degrees c.

Using a knife, carefully butterfly (slit through the centre) each chicken breast.

Lay chicken breasts flat on a cutting board and sprinkle with seasoned salt and Italian seasoning. Place 3 to 4 strips each of the string beans, carrots and red peppers. Sprinkle each with 2 tablespoons cheese.

Roll chicken breast up and place seam side down in a medium skillet.

Pour barbecue sauce over chicken and place in oven. Bake 20-25 minutes, basting with the barbecue sauce halfway through cooking.

Remove chicken breasts from pan. To serve, slice each breast into 4 or 5 slices, decorate in a fan shape. Pour a little extra barbeque sauce on the side.

Note: If barbeque sauce is not available, substitute with tomato-garlic sauce.

3 hi fibre cereal

Packed with goodness, this delicious cereal bowl is great with hot milk, or cold milk for that extra crunch.

Nutrients : vitamins B1, B2, B3, B5, E, folate, iron, magnesium, selenium, zinc

Preparation time : 5 minutes

Serves : 4

Ingredients :

- 8 tablespoons oats
- 2 tablespoons sesame seeds (roasted)
- 2 tablespoons sunflower seeds
- 2 tablespoons wheat flakes
- 2 tablespoons raisins
- 2 tablespoons chopped almonds
- 4 tablespoons barley flakes or bran
- Honey or maple syrup to taste (optional)

Directions : Mix the ingredients. Pour milk and serve.

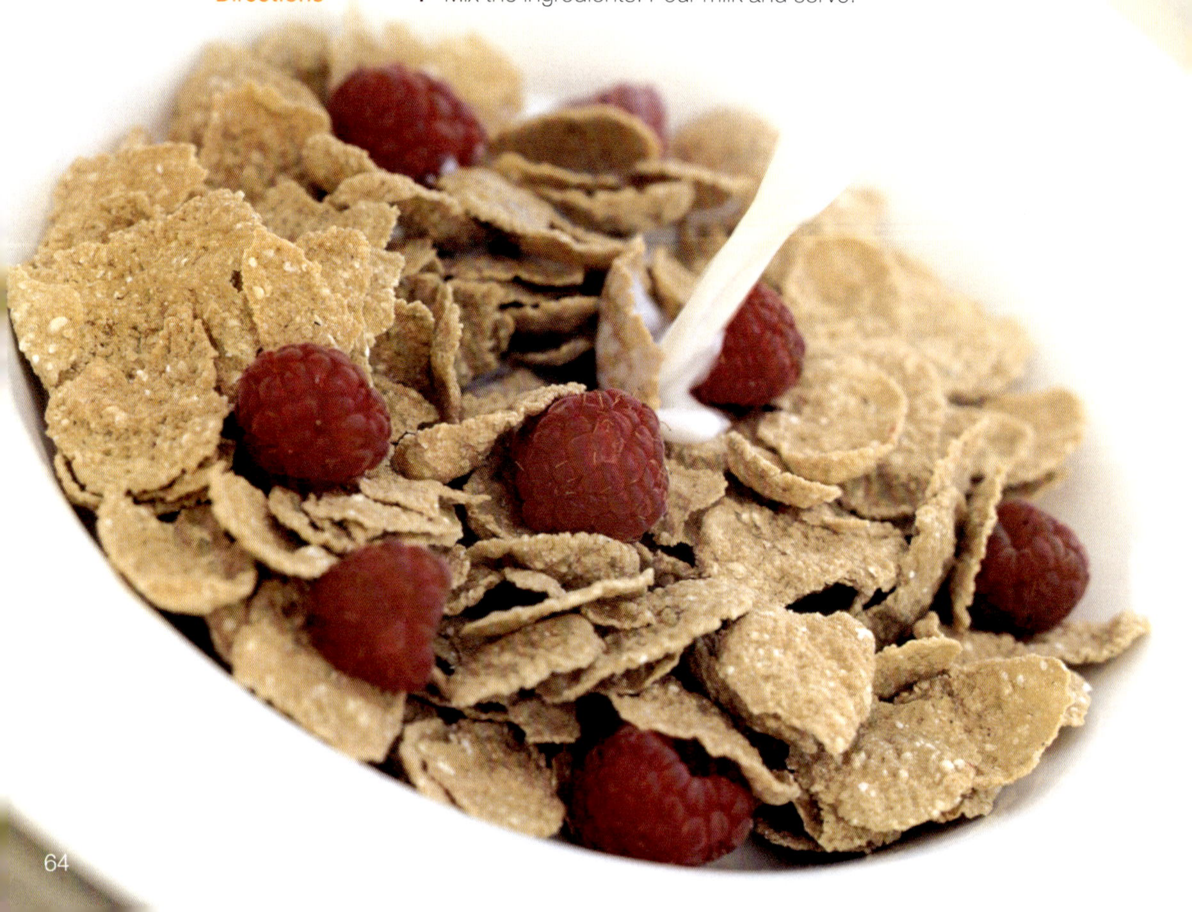

4 rainbow upma

A very unusual breakfast dish with dahlia instead of the regular semolina (rawa). The chopped veggies add colour of every hue, so it looks as appetizing as it tastes.

Nutrients : vitamin C, E, folate, iron, magnesium, zinc, protein, potassium, calcium

Preparation time : 20 minutes

Serves : 4

Ingredients :

2 cups roasted dahlia

1½ cups water

1 tablespoon oil

1 teaspoon mustard seeds

½ inch piece ginger, chopped fine

1 small onion, diced

1 small carrot, diced

½ capsicum, diced

½ cup corn kernels

1 floret cauliflower, diced

¼ cup coriander leaves

1 tablespoon lime juice

salt to taste

Directions :

Soak the dahlia in water for about ½ an hour.

Heat oil in a pan, add mustard seeds.

When mustard seeds splutter, add chopped ginger and onion. Stir for a minute.

Stir in all the remaining vegetables and keep on low flame till vegetables are cooked.

Drain the water from the dahlia and, along with the salt, mix with cooked vegetables.

Add 1½ cups water and cook until all the water is absorbed.

Sprinkle the lime juice on top and toss in the green coriander.

Mix well and serve hot.

5 legume spread on pita

This dish makes breakfast feel like a picnic. Your kids will enjoy the zesty flavours of vegetables and lemon, all served up on wholesome pita.

Nutrients : vitamin B2, B3, B5, B6, C, E, beta-carotene, folate, iron, lycopene

Preparation time : 15 minutes (Soaking time for chickpeas 6 hours)

Serves : 4

Ingredients :

4 pita breads (or 4 slices whole grain bread)
2 tablespoons chopped celery
1 tablespoon chopped spring onions
2 tablespoons chopped peppers (red, green, yellow)
1tablespoon sun dried tomatoes

For the legume spread

250 grams chickpeas
2 cloves garlic (crushed)
juice of 1 lemon
5 tablespoons thick fresh yoghurt
salt to taste

Directions : Cook the soaked chickpeas in a pressure cooker. Cool and drain. Add yoghurt, lemon juice, garlic and salt. Add water to get the desired consistency. Blend until mixture is smooth. Before serving add capsicum, celery, spring onions and red chili powder. Warm the pita bread, spread lettuce leaves, top with the spread and salad mixture.

6 fresh fruits with honey-yoghurt dressing

A healthier version of a fruit custard pudding, with honey instead of sugar.

Nutrients : calcium, potassium, fibre, zinc, protein, vitamin E

Preparation time : 10 minutes

Serves : 2

Ingredients :

1 large bowl cut fresh fruits
¼ cup mixed nuts
1 tablespoon sunflower seeds
1tablespoon raisins (soak for 10 minutes)

yoghurt-honey dressing

½ cup yoghurt (hung)
2 tablespoons honey

Directions : Mix the fruits, nuts, seeds and raisins. Add the mixed honey-yoghurt dressing.

7 egg salad

Boiled eggs never tasted so good! The tangy-cheesy fillings make this really delicious and you can keep varying the add-ons - try chopped celery or oregano flakes for a change.

Nutrients : protein, vitamins A, D, B 12, calcium, phosphorous, niacin

Preparation time : 15 minutes

Serves : 4

Ingredients :

- 6 hard boiled eggs, peeled
- 2 cubes softened cream cheese
- 1 tablespoon tomato sauce
- ¼ teaspoon pepper
- 1 sprig parsley / coriander, chopped fine
- salt to taste
- lettuce leaves

Directions :

Wet a sharp knife and cut the boiled eggs vertically. Carefully scoop out the yolk from all the eggs.

Mash the yolk and mix in the softened cream cheese and other ingredients.

Fill back this creamy mixture into the empty egg white cups. If you have an icing gun, you may use it to make patterns as you fill it in. Decorate with lettuce leaves, chill in the fridge for 20 minutes before serving.

FACT-O-Meter

Eggs are great for health and make a wholesome breakfast food. A medium-sized egg contains 6.5 grams of protein, 5.8 grams of fat and around 80 calories. It is loaded with vitamin A, vitamin D, and has the B 12 group of vitamins in abundance. Minerals in one egg include 29 mg of calcium, 103 mg phosphorous, and 6.2 mg magnesium.

Children can have 4 – 6 eggs a week. Their cholesterol intake should not exceed 300 mg a day. An egg typically contains 215 mg of cholesterol.

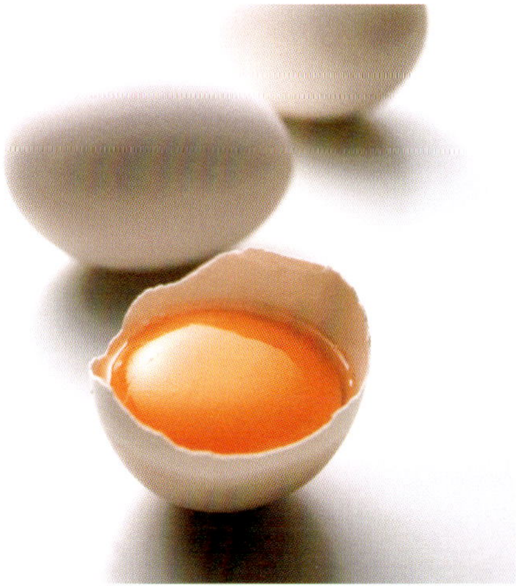

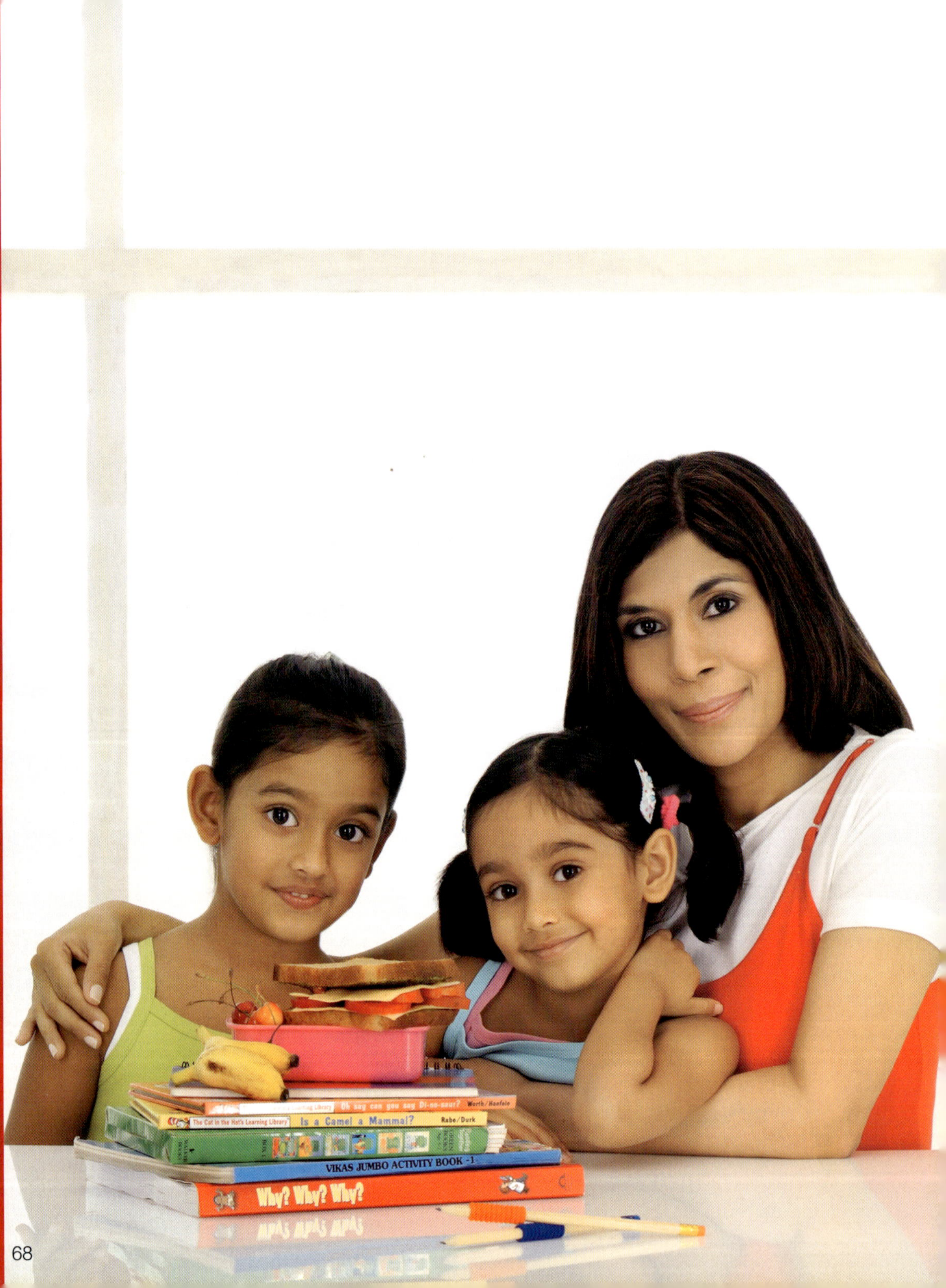
Oh say can you say Di-no-saur?
Worth/Haefele
The Cat in the Hat's Learning Library
Is a Camel a Mammal?
Rabe/Durk
VIKAS JUMBO ACTIVITY BOOK -1
Why? Why? Why?

Mantra 5

One-third of your child's daily nutrition comes from the **school lunch box.** It is therefore vital to pack in balanced, **easy-to-eat** meals, for **snacks,** the **main lunch,** even for the **bus trip** back home!

TIFFIN TIME-TABLE

School lunch menus and snack ideas can be a major dilemma. What should you pack? What is your child most likely to finish? Every time your child's lunch box comes home untouched, you probably blame yourself. I'm guessing you also worry about what got traded and what got thrown away. It's time to look for solutions. Give tiffins a new twist. Think out of the box. Entice your school-going child with tantalizing tiffin ideas.

Keep in mind, what a toddler at playschool enjoys isn't what a high school teenager can eat in front of friends! Depending on age, your child's individual preferences, your own family cooking traditions, and most important, your creative input, you can re-invent the tiffin box.

BEFORE WE DIVE INTO RECIPES, I WANT TO EMPHASIZE THAT CHILDREN CONSUME ONE-THIRD OF THEIR DAILY NOURISHMENT DURING SCHOOL HOURS. THE LUNCH BOX, THEREFORE, CANNOT BE TAKEN LIGHTLY!

- Most schools do not give much time for lunch. Snack breaks are also of a short duration. This limited time, for both lunch and snacks, is filled with distractions. So make sure the food is packed in easy-to-open packages, is easy to eat, and does not require peeling or special tools.
- Small children may not eat very much at one sitting. Think about packing appetizers instead of a large sandwich, which can be intimidating. Think mini idlis, or little sandwich triangles, baby carrots, or bite-size pieces of fruit. (Even spoons must be smaller!)
- If your child enjoys the same thing day after day, go ahead and pack it, as long as the overall meal is nutritious. Many kids don't like a lot of change in what they eat. Did you know that it takes 10 to 12 introductions to a new food before a child is usually willing to even taste it?
- Use an insulated thermos or tiffin box for hot foods like rice and dal, soup, or use the thermos for cold foods like salads or raita. For best results, rinse out the thermos with hot water before filling hot food. Similarly, rinse out with cold water for cold foods.
- Make your own snack mixes, with healthy additions like dried fruits, unsalted nuts, and baked crackers. Kids love to munch on something crunchy and sweet or savoury.
- For smaller kids, include something fun - a sticker, cookies wrapped in plastic wrap with a ribbon tie, sandwiches cut into playful shapes, or multicolored fruit and veggie combos.

As I have mentioned, lunch is an important meal. Five days a week, your child eats lunch in school. A healthy lunch box fuels your child's body and keeps the energy level up all afternoon. Improving the quality of lunch directly impacts your kid's school performance, for academics, as well as physical activity.

square meal

If children do not consume a proper lunch, they miss out on important nutrients so essential for their bodies and brains. To ensure your kids get all the important components for a balanced meal, think of a square lunch.

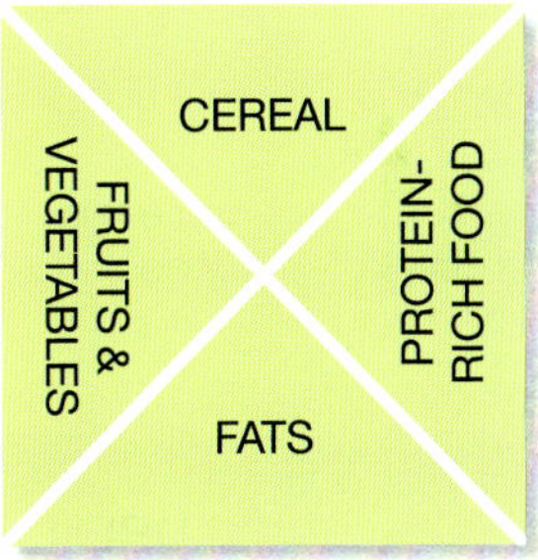

A SQUARE LUNCH INCLUDES THE 4 FOOD GROUPS

A balanced school lunch, comprising the 4 food groups, is vital. As with other meals, the lunch box too must follow the square meal concept. The 4 food groups include cereals, fruits and vegetables, protein-rich foods, and fats.

Start by getting your children involved in the planning process. Take your children shopping with you, at least once a month. Let them pick ingredients they like, from the cereals section, fruit and vegetable section, or a choice of lean protein-rich foods they prefer. Limit the ice-cream and avoid the packaged foods, especially processed meats and pizza and frozen ready-to-eat meals.

Apart from quality, keep an eye on quantity as well. Small portions are ideal, provided they are not too meagre and there is enough variety. A large quantity of one dish may not work – your child gets overwhelmed and doesn't know where to start!

PLAN FOR THE WEEK

Stock up ingredients for the week. This saves you precious time. You can also plan out an entire 5-day "tiffin time-table", with the help of your child. When you and your child mutually agree on an item, it becomes something to anticipate in the tiffin. If you have two kids, they can alternate weeks, or alternate days, to decide what goes in the lunch box. This way your kids also learn to be flexible about food.

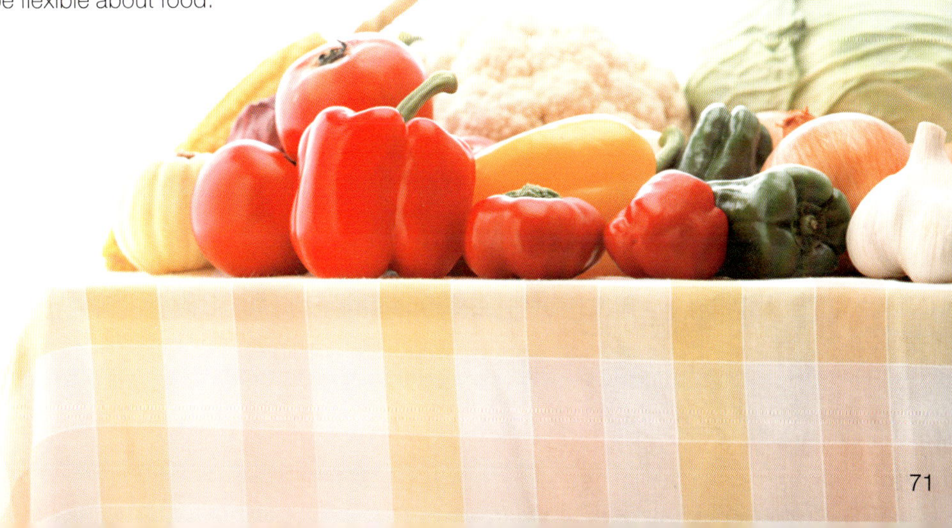

10 hot favourites on every kid's special request list

1. **wraps**
   Wrap and roll the school lunch! Roll up cheese, jams, vegetables, kebabs, spreads, peanut butter, anything your child likes, in a roti or pita. For older kids, consider wraps with paneer bhurji or spicy potato filling.

2. **sandwiches**
   The possibilities are endless. Lettuce and tomato, cheese, peanut butter, baked beans, paneer, chicken, fish, jams, it's a never-ending list of fillers you can experiment with. Stay with the options your child enjoys most.

3. **mini anything**
   Mini vegetable cutlets, kababs, patties, idlis, uttapam, you name it, your child will eat these bite-size items with relish.

4. **pizza pockets**
   A neat way to seal up drippy cheese-and-veggie or cheese-and-chicken fillings. Children love to bite into the gooey insides, while the pocket crust does not allow it to get messy.

5. **veggie 'hot dogs'**
   Make a simple vegetable sandwich with a long patty using a hot dog bun instead of regular bread.

6. **stir fry veggies in rice**
   This is best for older kids. Very versatile as stir fried rice, a veggie pulao, or even a chicken hot pot.

7. **cold pasta salad**
   A yummy summer lunch dish. With assorted pasta shapes for visual appeal, seasonal veggies, and a cheesy sauce to top it all, it's an all-time lunch box favourite.

8. **idli sandwich**
   A delectable twist to the traditional idli . The steamed idlis become a sandwich with fillings like cream cheese, mint chutney, even salsa or tomato sauce.

9. **stuffed parathas**
   The lunch that packs a punch! Stuff the paratha with your child's favourite veggies, grated paneer, cheese, corn, mutton mince, or the perennially popular potato.

10. **bhel & chaat box**
    It sounds so decadent, your child will love it! But this is a healthy version, and will be a hit with you and your child! Made with crunchy moong sprouts, potato, a bit of sev, and a rich tamarind date chutney (to be packed in a separate mini container, so the chaat ingredients don't go soggy), it's a real treat for chaat lovers.

Do other kids envy your child's lunch?

Many of you Moms would be taking a lot of trouble to make the lunch box super special. Tinku's Mom Tina was one such Mom. Tinku, a third grader, loved his lunch, but guess what? As soon as he opened his dabba, other kids came by to check it out.

By the time Tinku got any food, there was very little left! His Mom wondered why, in spite of the lunch box being empty, Tinku came back home so ravenous.

At first she thought he was discarding the entire lunch. Then, after some probing, she discovered what was really happening. So Tina put a simple plan in place. She bought a 2-tiered lunch box. One section was labeled "Tinku". The other section was labeled "friends". She packed adequate amounts of food in both sections.

This way the other school kids understood that Tinku had to finish his own lunch. At the same time, they also felt included!

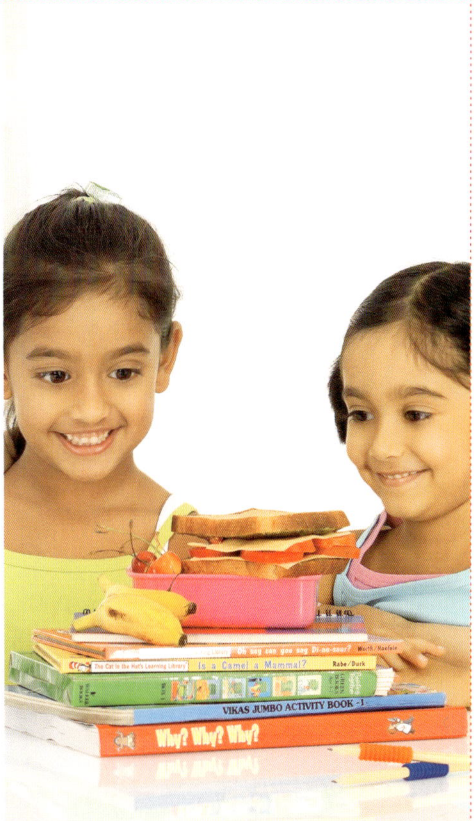

SCHOOL CAFETERIA VERSUS HOME LUNCH

As kids get older, they want to try out the school cafeteria. Some of their peers probably order school lunch on a daily basis and the glamour of restaurant-style eating has its attractions!

Don't ban it altogether. Let them occasionally spend their money in the school cafeteria. Today, most schools offer healthier options, apart from the samosa and paratha menus.

Once they try it out a few times, the kids tire of the same old "canteen" taste, and are happy to make it an occasional habit. Also, if your home food is nicely packaged, with tasty, tempting options, they will come right back to it.

FOOD SWAPPING

We all did it! Kids are naturally curious, so they will always want to try out some treat in a friend's dabba. They also love sharing, and in itself, that is a good thing. What you can do is tell them to eat a little bit of everything from their own tiffin, before they start handing it around.

types of tiffins

stainless steel carriers

+ This is like unpacking a stacked thali! All the different items - dal-rice, roti, vegetable and curds – are the staples that make up a balanced thali. Kids would be getting a hygienic, home-cooked lunch with all the food groups included.

- The only drawback is that kids may not have the time to finish it. If they do manage to consume the entire lunch, it may be too heavy, making them sleepy in the afternoon. An option could be to pack either roti, or rice, not both.

thermos containers

+ A great way to pack hot or cold food. Particularly convenient for wet food like pasta, soup, rice, or noodles. Cold options like salads and chaats stay fresh and unspoiled. This can often be served up as a one-dish meal - all it takes is to dig in and enjoy.

- Can get a little messy. May not be the ideal option for very small kids.

plastic boxes / insulated boxes

+ Best for dry lunches, such as sandwiches and wraps. The great thing is, you can stuff smaller boxes in these main boxes, for extras like raita, or dessert. Ensure you buy food grade plastic, so there is no unpleasant "plasticky" smell to the food.

- Not practical for wet food, as it can leak. This restricts the kind of dishes you can pack.

brown paper bags

+ Good for certain types of dry snacks. Eco-friendly and convenient, as they can be dumped at school, and there is no empty dabba to carry home.

- Kids tend to crush the food in their school bags. Not an option for wet food.

Depending on what you are packing for lunch, you can vary the containers every day. Try to keep the snack-time foods separate, so that your child does not mix it up with the main lunch meal.

Always pack tissues or wet wipes along with the tiffin. Some parents even pack in a hand sanitizer spray. If your children never seem to remember to wash their hands before eating their school lunch, this is the solution!

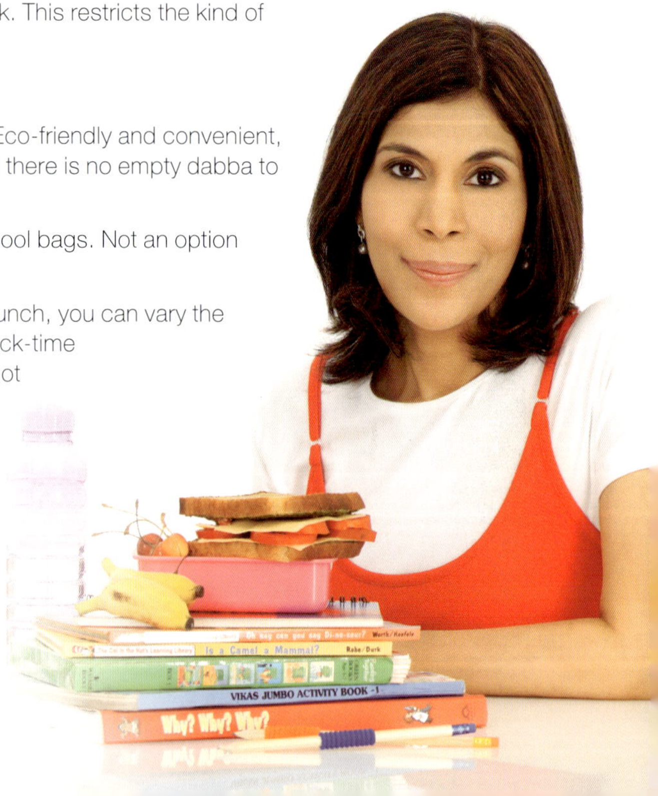

sample lunch boxes, with a 2-week time-table

My lunch menu schedule helps you get organized, keeps it simple, and guarantees very nutritious lunch options. When you offer different foods throughout the week, not only are you providing varied nutrients, but also helping kids to appreciate and enjoy a range of foods.

I have suggested you pack in a treat as a device to entice your child to open the lunch box. It can be anything that your child enjoys and looks forward to. Yet, as you will see, it can also be nutritious!

In the 2-week tiffin time-tables that follow, I have devised a balanced meal plan for the snack recess as well as the main lunch.

You will also find the main lunch menus are square meals in themselves, all including the 4 essential food groups – cereal, fruits and veggies, protein-rich food and fat. Try to follow the same "square meal" principle for all 5 days of the week.

To further cater to your child's nutritional needs, you could aim for one lunch each week that helps to boost brain power, one to provide good energy and one that the kids get to pick. Also be sure to include a picnic type lunch that is easy to do, but is also heart-healthy. Finally, include a lunch that is easy on you, quick to make, but still a healthy option.

WEEK ONE LUNCH BOX

SNACK	SQUARE MEAL LUNCH	DESSERT	BENEFITS
MONDAY dates & almonds crackers	cottage cheese roll / tuna fish salad roll	banana stuffed with peanut butter	brain food
TUESDAY fruit salad	vegetable pulao / chicken pulao	kurmura chikki	energy booster
WEDNESDAY yoghurt cup carrot & cucumber sticks	macaroni & cheese with veggies	fig barfi / kaju katli	kids pick
THURSDAY peanut kurmura mix	tandoori chicken roti wrap/ tandoori paneer tikka wrap	whole wheat halwa	protein power
FRIDAY trail mix apple	tomato cheese sandwich/ chicken sandwich	chocolate milk	super-fast express

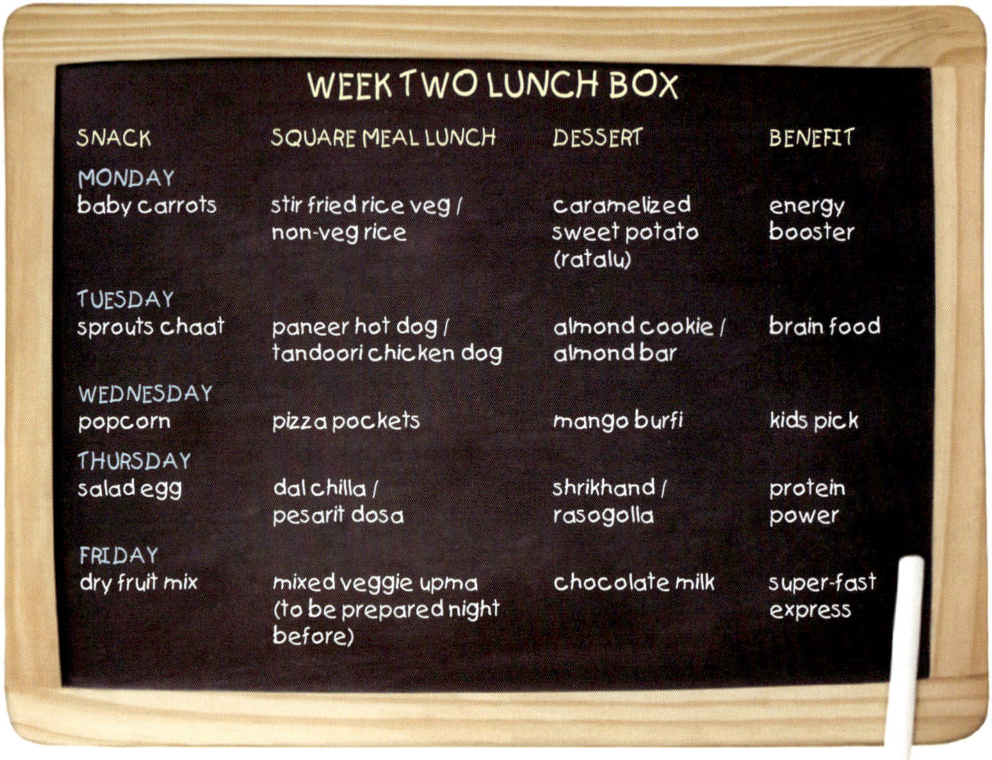

WEEK TWO LUNCH BOX

SNACK	SQUARE MEAL LUNCH	DESSERT	BENEFIT
MONDAY baby carrots	stir fried rice veg / non-veg rice	caramelized sweet potato (ratalu)	energy booster
TUESDAY sprouts chaat	paneer hot dog / tandoori chicken dog	almond cookie / almond bar	brain food
WEDNESDAY popcorn	pizza pockets	mango burfi	kids pick
THURSDAY salad egg	dal chilla / pesarit dosa	shrikhand / rasogolla	protein power
FRIDAY dry fruit mix	mixed veggie upma (to be prepared night before)	chocolate milk	super-fast express

DELICIOUS, NUTRITIOUS TIFFIN LUNCH RECIPES

1 tuna roll

Serves : 4 rolls

Ingredients :
- 200 gm. tinned tuna
- ¼ cup assorted veggies - onion, celery, olives, chopped fine
- 1 tablespoon mayonnaise
- ½ tablespoon tomato ketchup
- pinch pepper
- chili flakes (for older kids)
- 4 whole wheat bread rolls

Directions : Mix all the ingredients well. Split the bread roll into half, fill with tuna mixture. Secure the stuffed roll in plastic cling wrap.

2 pulao veg / non-veg

Serves : 4 portions

Ingredients : 4 cups basmati rice, semi-cooked

2 teaspoons ginger-garlic paste

4 onions, chopped

4 tablespoon cooking oil

2 cups water

1 cup mixed veggies like carrots, French beans, tinda, cauliflower,cut into big pieces *

4 teaspoons tomato paste

2 teaspoons jeera-dhania powder

½ teaspoon haldi

1 teaspoon chili powder

½ teaspoon garam masala powder

salt to taste

* substitute veggies with chicken pieces to make non-veg pulao

Directions : Heat the oil in a thick-bottomed utensil. Add the ginger garlic paste, brown lightly. Add chopped onions, cook until transparent. Add the chopped vegetables along with the powdered masalas, tomato paste, and salt to taste.

When the vegetables brown slightly, add ½ cup water. Let the water evaporate. Then add the semi-cooked rice with the remained 1 ½ cups water. Cook covered, until water dries up.

While packing, you will have to mix the vegetables from the bottom with the rice on top.

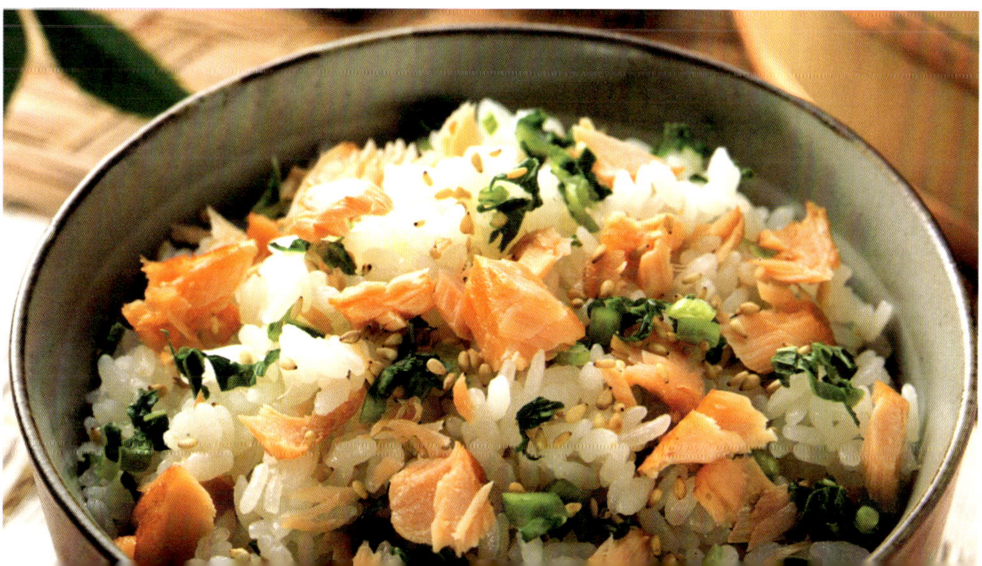

3 macaroni'n cheese

Serves : 4

Ingredients : 2 cups whole wheat elbow macaroni, cooked

1 cup mixed carrots, French beans, zucchini and peppers, cooked

1 small onion, chopped fine

for the sauce

1 small stick butter

1 cup milk

2 tablespoons whole wheat flour (or maida)

½ cup cheddar cheese, grated

½ teaspoon pepper

½ teaspoon jeera powder (optional)

2 tablespoons tomato paste

Directions : Melt the stick of butter in a hot pan. Add chopped onion. After 2 minutes, add the whole wheat flour, mix well to avoid lumps. Add the milk and stir constantly. Then add the chopped vegetables.

Mix in the grated cheese, tomato paste, seasonings and cooked pasta. Combine all ingredients well. Cook till the sauce is of a semi-liquid consistency, then remove from fire. This sauce will thicken as it cools.

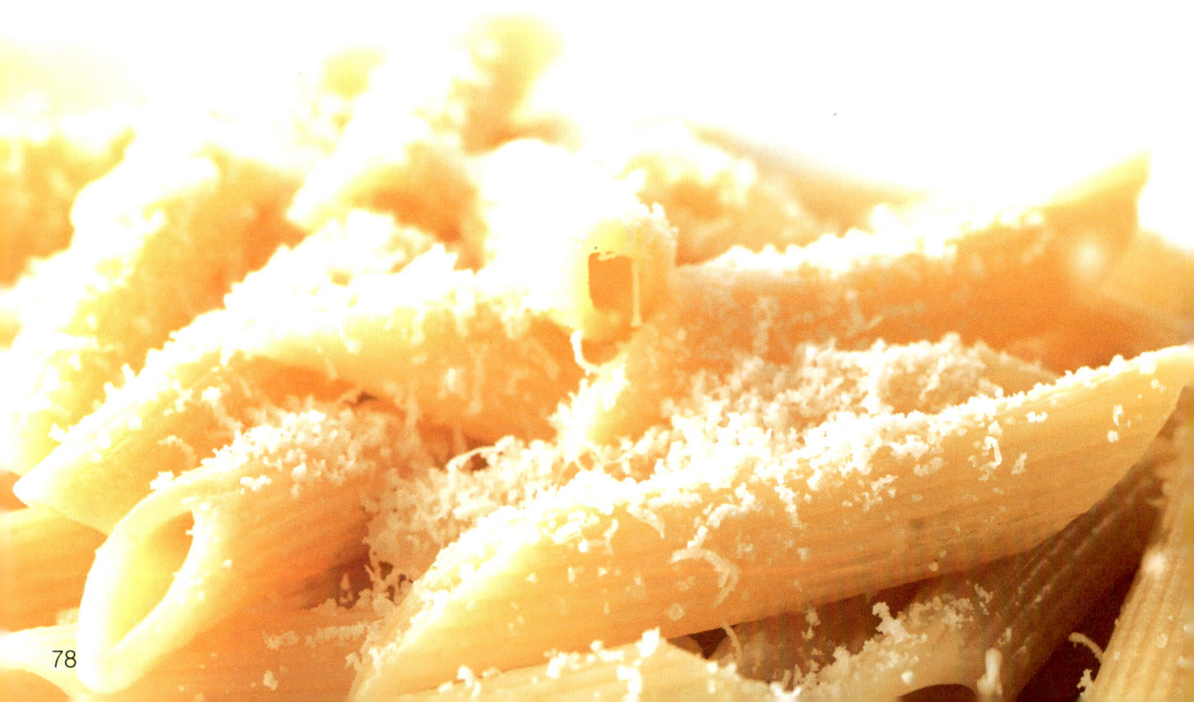

4 roti wrap veg /non-veg

Serves : 2

Ingredients : 4 rotis

16 cubes tandoori paneer *

¼ cup green onion, chopped fine

¼ cup green coriander, chopped fine

½ teaspoon chaat masala

½ teaspoon chili powder (for older kids)

* Substitute the tandoori paneer with tandoori chicken for non-veg option.

Directions : Lay out a roti flat, and fill with 4 tandoori paneer cubes. Sprinkle the masalas and top with chopped onion and coriander. Roll up the roti tightly and secure in tin foil. Make sure the two ends are properly sealed.

5 moong dal chilla / pesarit dosa

Serves : 2

Ingredients : 1 cup whole moong dal, soaked overnight

1" ginger, peeled and chopped fine

1-2 small green chillies, chopped fine

¼ teaspoon turmeric

¼ teaspoon asafoetida (hing)

1 small onion, chopped fine

2 tablespoons coriander, chopped fine

oil for frying

salt to taste

Directions : Grind the moong dal with ½ cup water, into a coarse paste. Add chopped ginger, garlic, chillies, asafoetida and turmeric. Season to taste.

Pour batter into a bowl and add chopped onion and coriander. Mix well.

Heat a teaspoon of oil in a pan. Drop a ladleful of batter in the centre of the pan. Using the back of the ladle spread the batter into a circle. Make sure the chilla is not too thick so it gets cooked evenly.

Add a little oil along the edges of the chilla, cover and cook for 2 minutes. Turn the chilla over and cook on the other side until it becomes golden brown.

Pack with a piece of jaggery or coconut chutney.

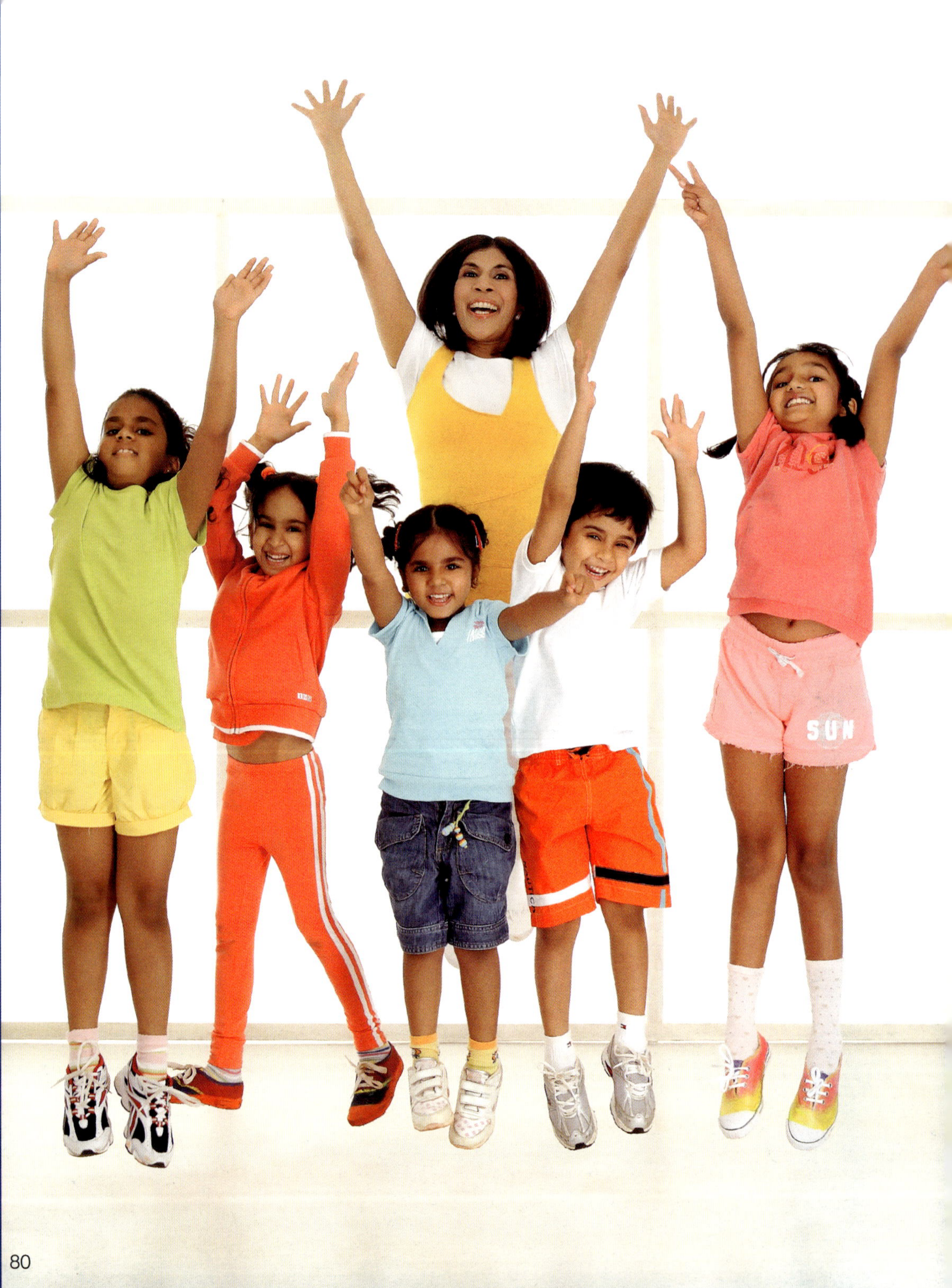

Mantra 6

Fitness is a state of mind. The **Jaldi Fit Quiz** in this chapter **evaluates** your child's **inclination** and **attitude** towards various forms of **exercise.**

JALDI FIT CHIDREN'S QUIZ

Take the Jaldi Fit Quiz to evaluate your child's fitness attitude. This evaluation serves as a basic tool to tweak your children's daily habits, to optimize their health and energy.

READ THE 5 POINTS BELOW, THEN ANSWER WITH A CLEAR 'YES' OR 'NO'.

- my child is regular with exercise Yes ☐ No ☐
- my child enjoys "time out" spent in physical activity Yes ☐ No ☐
- exercise improves my child's mood Yes ☐ No ☐
- my child is willing to balance television time with play time Yes ☐ No ☐
- my child is open to trying newer forms of physical activity Yes ☐ No ☐

If you've answered "Yes" to at least 4 of them, your child has the right fitness attitude. If 2 or more questions have a "NO" answer, you have work to do. However, there is no cause for worry, as this section specifically guides you towards result-oriented solutions.

FAMILY FITNESS

A child who has active parents is six times more likely to be physically active. Children learn by example. Set a good example by exercising regularly yourself. On weekends you can go together to the park or to the swimming pool, as a family. A little friendly competition can be fun - don't be surprised if your 9-year old son beats you!

BENEFITS OF EXERCISE

- reduces risk of heart disease and other ailments
- improves sleep patterns
- keeps the body strong and in-shape
- boosts energy levels
- improves posture
- helps concentration
- reduces stress and anxiety
- enhances self esteem

assess your child's fitness personality

Each child's fitness personality is unique. Take a few moments to jot down your child's fitness personality. Remember, inactive children are likely to become inactive adults. Physical activity produces overall physical, psychological and social benefits.

1. is your child athletic or active?
2. is your child a casual athlete?
3. is your child non-athletic or sedentary?

An **athletic or active** child will want to be on the basketball team or excel in swimming; while the **casual athlete** may just enjoy playing cricket or badminton in the playground. The **non-athletic** child, on the other hand, is likely to need a parent's help and encouragement to get physically active.

THE ACTIVE & ATHLETIC CHILD

Your child is committed to a sport or regular physical activity, and is likely to concentrate on practice time. You child also enjoys the thrill of competition. Teach your kid that it's not only about winning, but the joy of engaging in a sport or exercise is important too.

An enduring passion for a sport or exercise is a sure way of ensuring continued interest into adulthood. Good going. Keep it up!

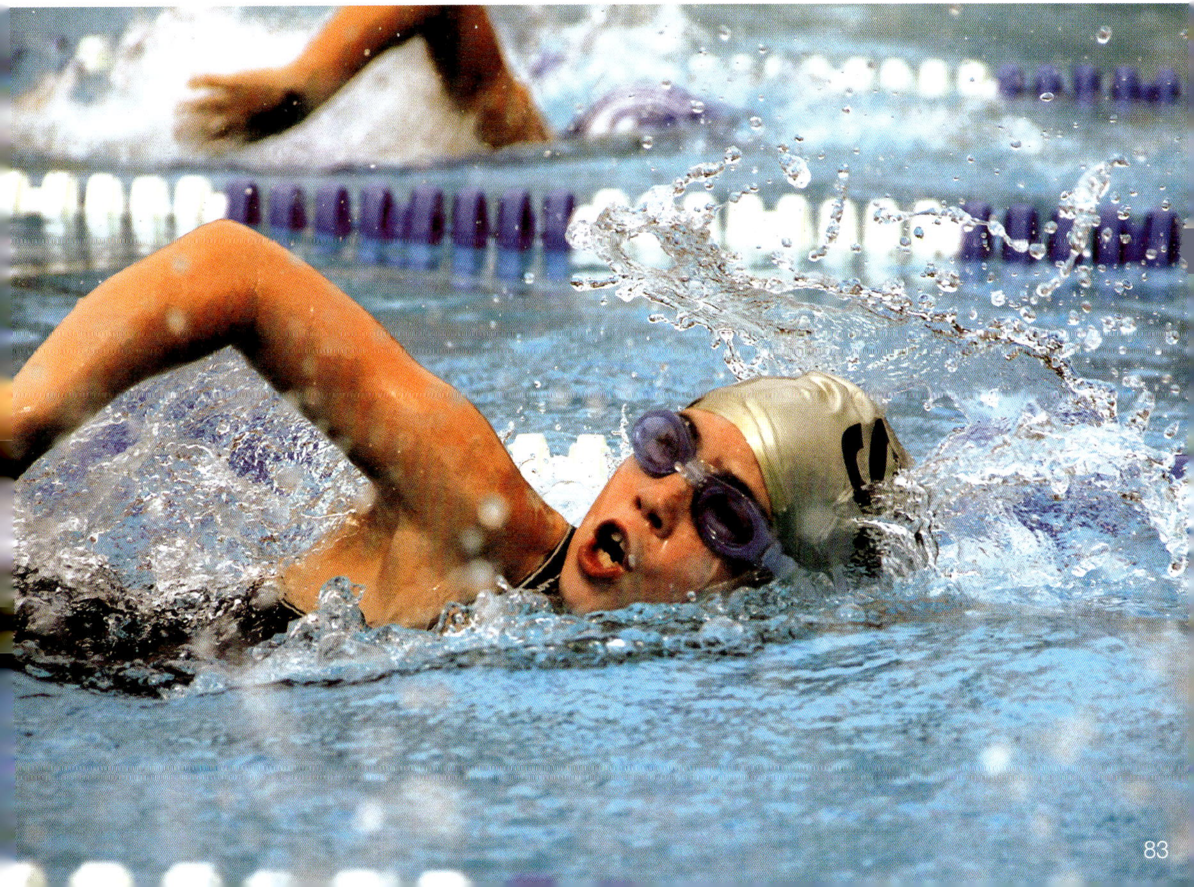

RECOMMENDATIONS

- ✓ help him / her remain focused and motivated
- ✓ encourage your child to constantly improve skills and remain challenged
- ✓ evaluate progress
- ✓ encourage participation in sports
- ✓ watch as many professional matches as possible with your child

FIT Tip

Support efforts and also check that your child:

- manages schoolwork
- gets enough rest and sleep

Children who take up a strenuous endurance sport, like tennis, cricket, running, or competitive swimming, need to consume greater quantities of food to sustain their energy levels. This is because these sports often involve 1½ to over 2 hours of continuous physical activity, testing a child's stamina to the limit.

Ensure your children are able to cope with the enormous demand on their energy and endurance - give them a diet that gears them to perform at optimum capacity.

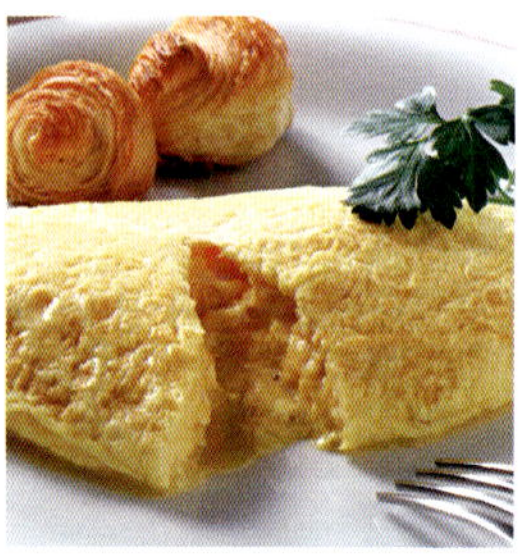

PROTEINS

Protein is needed to build and repair muscles. Protein-rich foods include fish and poultry, dairy products, nuts and soya products. Adequate nourishment and regular training help to build strong, sturdy muscles.

Caution Too much protein can lead to dehydration and calcium loss. Therefore, protein supplements, if required, should be prescribed by your child's nutritionist.

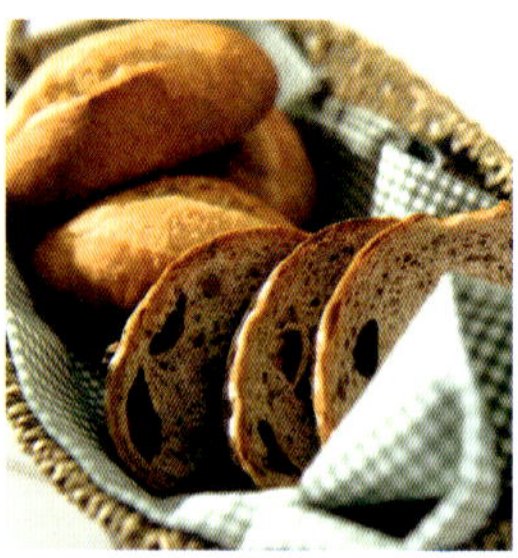

CARBOHYDRATES

Carbs provide the body with energy. When you are planning your child's meals, look for unprocessed, fibre-rich carbohydrates, like whole-wheat pasta, brown rice, wholegrain bread and cereal. Make sure your child consumes plenty of fruits and vegetables.

For more information on nutrition, visit www.liveactive.com

SNACK SUGGESTIONS

A healthy snack for active children can include yoghurt and banana, wholegrain cereal and milk, cottage cheese or chicken sandwich, mixed dried fruits and nuts.

drink up!

It's important for young athletes to drink plenty of fluids to prevent dehydration, which can zap strength, energy, and coordination and lead to heat-related illness. Even mild dehydration can affect athletic performance.

Thirst is not a reliable indicator of hydration status. Experts recommend that kids drink water or other fluids every 15 to 20 minutes during physical activity. Fluids must also be consumed after the activity is over, to re-hydrate the body.

Although many sports drinks are available, plain water is usually enough to keep kids hydrated. Sports drinks are designed to provide energy and replace electrolytes - such as sodium and potassium - that athletes lose in sweat.

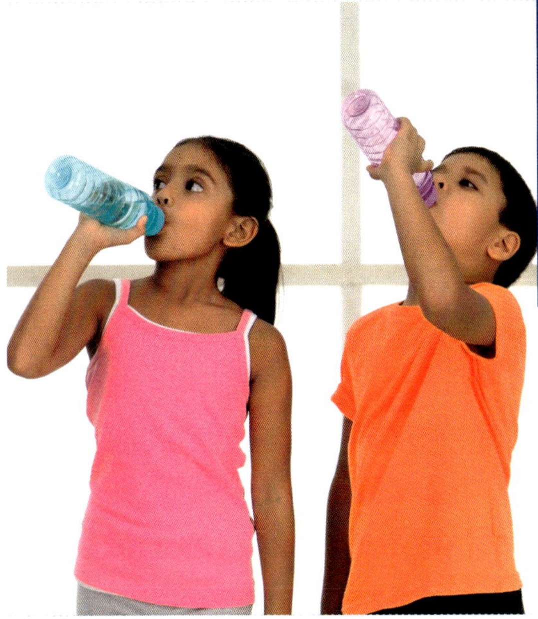

THE CASUAL ATHLETE

Your child likes being active, but may not be driven enough to participate in competitive sports. Most children fall in this category. They are perfectly happy and fit – being casual participants.

While your child has fairly good exercise habits, some activities can be better channeled. Expose your child to different types of sports and physical activities. This way you may discover an interest or talent in some sport. Encourage small changes that can make a big difference to improving health.

RECOMMENDATIONS

- ✔ evaluate your child's fitness habits and set achievable goals
- ✔ aim to fit in exercise 5 to 7 days a week
- ✔ reward, praise and offer encouragement
- ✔ vary physical activity routines

FIT Tip

- maintain focused attention during practice and watch your game or sport improve
- motivation is a crucial factor in any exercise regimen. Without motivation, it is all too easy to make excuses to slack off. Slacking off for a day can turn into slacking off for a week, a month, and eventually quitting the fitness habit altogether

PRACTICE MAKES PERFECT

Deepak, like many casual athletes, swam for pleasure. He loved playing and splashing about in the water. His proficiency in the pool gave Deepak a chance to participate in the school's blue house swimming team. But he was too lazy to practice regularly. He took part in his school swimming competition and lost the event.

Deepak was deeply disappointed and wished he had tried a little harder to make the cut. The following year, Deepak was determined to win the school swimming trophy - with a dedicated, never-say-die attitude, he did!

THE NON-ATHLETIC OR SEDENTARY CHILD

Your child may lack interest in physical activity. Long hours on the computer or addiction to the television can result in a sedentary lifestyle. Finding a fun activity for your child can be the motivating factor that leads to a lifetime of physical fitness.

Use this evaluation as a turning point. Address areas that need to be improved tactfully.

RECOMMENDATIONS

- ✔ encourage physical activity based on your child's personality
- ✔ educate your child to recognize the fact that exercise will improve performance at school and play
- ✔ set times for homework, play and exercise
- ✔ make exercise time a fun time. Join in! Play games, walk, take a trip to the park or play a sport
- ✔ praise your child's efforts

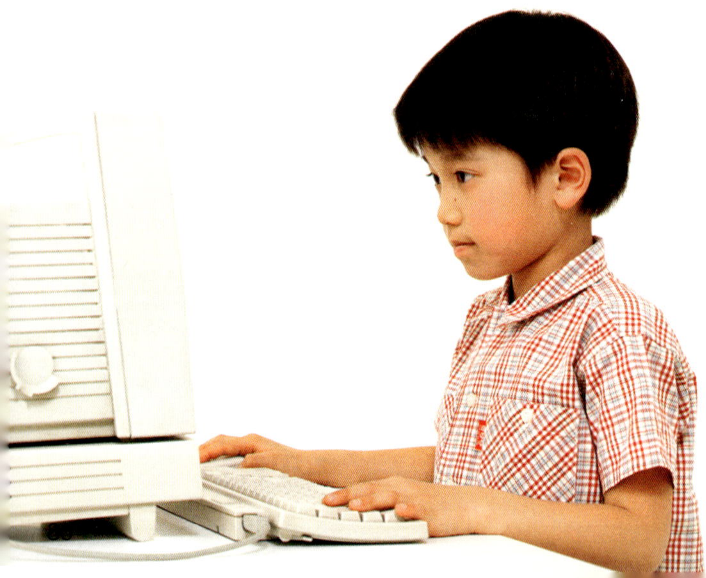

PARENT **ALERT!**

You can encourage, inspire, and equip your child's activity. Help by providing the sports gear, taking care of transportation, and above all, participating as a role model!

- allot time
- be regular
- set goals
- maintain a log
- review
- reward

fitness assessments

As children grow older, they may be inclined to take on more physically challenging activities. Fitness assessments make it possible to measure improvements. Re-test after 6 weeks to track progress.

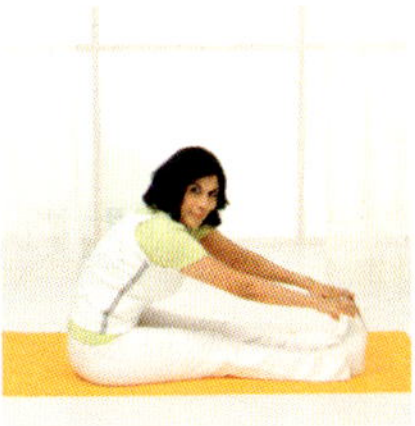

How flexible is your child?

TEST YOUR CHILD: Ask your child to sit on the floor, back against a wall and legs joined together, extended in front. Make your child reach forward, as far out as possible. Measure how far out your child's fingertips can reach.

a. Thighs b. Knee c. Shin and beyond

This test measures leg and lower back flexibility.

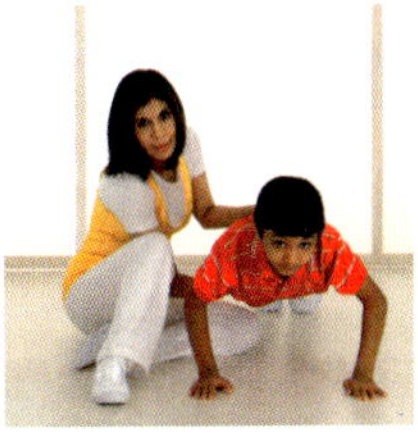

How powerful is your child's upper body?

TEST YOUR CHILD: This push-up test measures the strength and endurance of the upper body. Boys should use the standard "military style" push-up position with only the hands and the toes touching the floor. Girls have the option of using the "bent knee" position. To do this, girls must kneel on the floor, hands on either side of the chest, back straight.

This test measures the strength and endurance of the upper body and is important in maintaining good posture. The objective of this test is to complete as many push-ups as possible at a constant pace.

Make your child do as many push-ups as possible in one minute. Record the number.

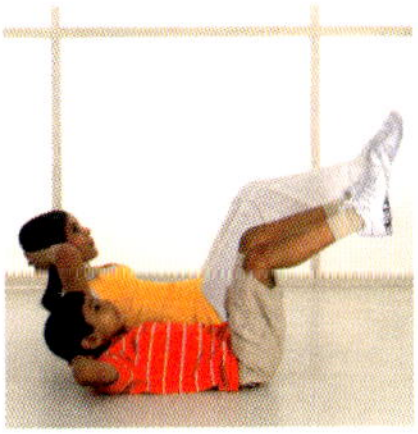

How strong are your child's abdominals?

TEST YOUR CHILD: The abs crunch test measures the strength and endurance of the abdominals and hip-flexor muscles. Get your child to lie on a carpeted or cushioned floor with feet flat on the ground, knees bent approximately at right angles.

Ask your child to lie on the back with hands placed behind the head. Bend knees at a 90 degree angle, and raise shoulders, to feel the ab muscles contract, then lower.

Make your child do as many crunches as possible in one minute. Record the number.

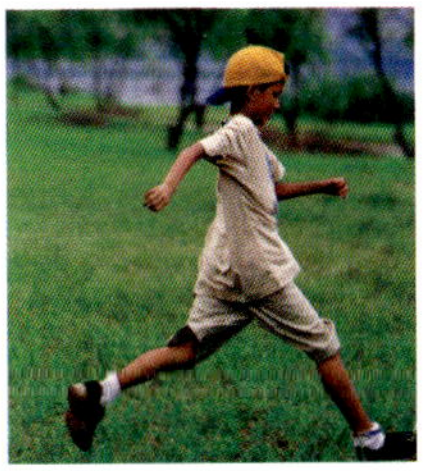

How good is your child's speed?

TEST YOUR CHILD: Get your child to run 500 metres (younger children can be given shorter distances) and note the time.

This is perhaps the most important indicator of physical fitness, as it assesses the capacity of the cardiovascular system by measuring speed and stamina.

Q: My child needs to gain weight, should he exercise?

A: Yes, exercise has numerous benefits. It is important to eat adequate nutritious food and exercise regularly to improve stamina, strength, keep fit and healthy. Exercise also improves appetite.

Q: Is PE (physical education) at school adequate?

A: No. The PE lessons offered in schools are rarely adequate. At least one hour of exercise per day is recommended. At present, most schools do not offer a daily PE routine of one hour. In fact, within the limited time allocated, changing clothes, lining up and getting instructions take up a substantial portion of time, further reducing the actual time spent on physical activity.

raising a fit kid

The goal is not always to produce a super athlete, but to raise a child who loves being active and is happy to run, exercise and play.

PRESCHOOLERS (4-5 YEARS)

Good habits are best started early. A child at age 4 is instinctively active – develop this instinct. Take your child to the park, playground, encourage learning of basic sporting skills such as throwing and kicking the ball, skipping, jumping, running and pedaling a tricycle or a bicycle. Unstructured exercise doesn't require any lessons. It's what children do naturally when given the opportunity to be active.

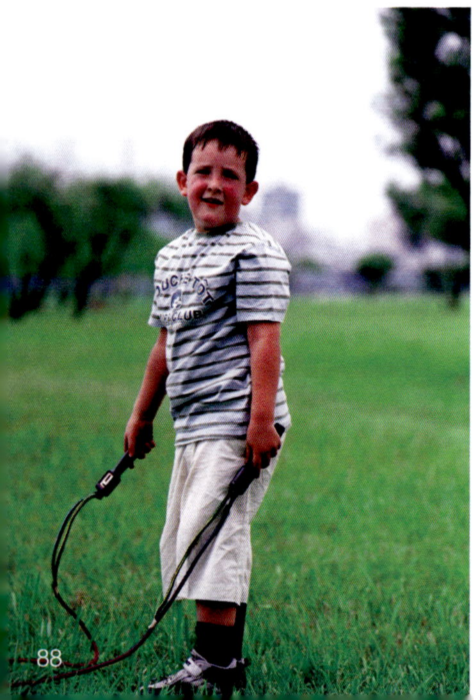

SCHOOL-AGE CHILDREN (6-12 YEARS)

By the age of 6 or 7 children are physically better equipped to participate in sports. They have longer attention spans and begin to grasp rules. While some children are motivated by competitive play, many are not ready for the increased pressure until 10 or 11 years of age.

This is a good age to develop hand-eye coordination and a basic understanding of rules for games and sports. Moderate-intensity activities can include swimming, bicycling, team sports and outdoor play. Many kids prefer to start with non-competitive sports and opt for competitive sports as they become older.

Research indicates that children above 10 years of age are more likely to participate in mentally and physically challenging activities. They might want to focus on an organized sport, develop specific skills and grasp complex strategies. Remember, too, that with competitive sport, your child's attitude must remain positive, with losses and setbacks taken in a sportsmanlike spirit.

As a child grows older, take into account his or her interests, temperament and body type. A mild-mannered boy may not prefer rugby, but may enjoy the challenge of tennis. Likewise, a girl may prefer ballet, or yoga, rather than a fast-paced sport like soccer. You can present your children with varied fitness options and offer advice. But ultimately, they must decide based on their personal preferences, because they have to enjoy what they do in the long run.

ADOLESCENTS (13 + YEARS)

By the time they reach age thirteen, less than half of all teenagers get regular exercise.

Whenever Madhu said to her two boys, "It's such a beautiful day, why don't you go for a swim?" the boys grumbled, "Mom is always telling us what to do." Whether they complied with the suggestion or continued to sprawl in front of the television set, is immaterial. The point is, parents cannot dictate how teenagers must spend their leisure time!

The teens are a period when kids want to be seen making independent choices. As their bodies change, they gain height and strength, your children are growing into young adults.

It therefore makes more sense to interact, rather than expect them to blindly follow instructions. Talk about the benefits of exercise, encourage your teenager to be an active, mature and independent individual. From the start of the discussion, make sure you discuss what is practical, feasible and affordable, from your point of view. This leaves no room for argument at a later stage.

I have to acknowledge that getting your teenager's attention may not be easy! The technology-loving teenager of today, with one hand on mobile text messaging and one eye on the e-mail, can hardly be enthusiastic about hours of physical activity.

But the fact of the matter is, teenagers need to be exercising just as much as they did when they were younger. They need time to be "unwired" so they don't become inactive adults. Whether it is running, competitive sports, gymnastics, or bicycling, encourage your teenage child to fit in fitness.

watch out!

In adolescence, girls could develop an eating disorder called anorexia nervosa. This can result in behavioral symptoms such as under-eating or over-exercising, or a combination of both. Mostly girls at this age strive to be too thin. The media - showcasing fashion icons and celebrities – often promotes the message that thin bodies are desirable. Hollywood and Bollywood set impossible standards, making teenage girls believe that, in order to be attractive, they need to be skinny.

When teenage girls exercise too much, or put themselves on a severely restricted diet, they are putting themselves at risk for serious health problems. This could then become an obsession that requires medical intervention.

WHAT YOU CAN DO

1. suggest counseling to stop self-destructive behaviour
2. emphasise the importance of being healthy and fit
3. help them set realistic and reasonable goals

ACTIVITY CHART

AGE	FOR DEVELOPMENT	SUGGESTED TIME
Pre-Schoolers		
4 - 5 Years	Playing outdoors, using push or pull toys, walking, running, jumping, kicking, bouncing the ball.	1½ to 2hrs
School-Age Children		
6 - 12 Years	Hand-eye coordination, building skills such as skipping rope, learning a sport, outdoor play.	1½ to 2hrs
Adolescents		
13 + Years	Choose according to interest, play team or individual sports.	30 to 60 minutes

IMPORTANCE OF SLEEP AND REST

Sleep requirements can vary between seven to ten hours, depending on your child's needs. Get your child into the habit of going to sleep and waking up at the same time each day so that the body adjusts to a regular sleeping pattern. Children who keep odd hours tend to toss and turn at night, not allowing themselves a restful night's sleep.

This affects their performance and efficiency in the day-time, because, without sleep, the mind and body cannot function optimally. Lack of sleep can also lead to lowered immunity, resulting in illness.

EXAM TIME

Even during exams, you can allocate at least 20 to 30 minutes for exercise. In fact, exercise is a great stress-buster and also improves concentration. If your child uses just this little bit of time to move around and be active, blood circulation improves. It becomes much easier to sit for the long exam hours with a clear head and a steady hand.

Mithun, a 14-year old boy says, "I always go for a 20-minute run or go cycling before I study in the evening. This really wakes me up and leaves me feeling energized so I can hit the books with some power!"

breaking the barriers

BARRIER 1: NOT ENOUGH TIME TO EXERCISE

Setting aside time to exercise can be a challenge. Planning is the key. For example, Monday through Friday, your kids can play with friends after school. Weekends is a good time for you to get involved, by taking the kids to the pool, or for a bike ride.

BARRIER 2: EXERCISE IS BORING

Choose activities your children enjoy. Remember, anything that gets them moving counts as exercise. Rotate different activities, such as playing football, swimming, cycling, and in the case of smaller children, taking them to the park to try out the swings, slides and jungle gym.

BARRIER 3: MY CHILD IS SELF-CONSCIOUS BECAUSE SHE IS OUT OF SHAPE

Overweight children do tend to be more self-conscious. Talking to your child will instill a feeling of self-confidence. If a child is uncomfortable exercising in the presence of others, exercising solo is an option. Then, as fitness levels improve and the child becomes more comfortable with exercise, group fitness activities can be considered.

BARRIER 4: MY CHILD IS TOO TIRED TO EXERCISE

It's a vicious cycle. If children do not exercise, energy levels will simply not pick up. It is therefore important to break the inertia. Only regular physical activity can give children the energy boost that helps them stay active.

BARRIER 5: MY CHILD IS NOT ATHLETIC

Natural athletic ability isn't a prerequisite to physical activity. Get your child to try something simple, something he or she can sustain on a regular basis. An option could be playing cricket in the building compound, with neighbourhood friends. Team workouts or sports generate loads of positive, goal oriented-energy. The idea is to have fun while exercising, without worrying about becoming a sports superstar!

For more exercise tips, log onto my website www.liveactive.com

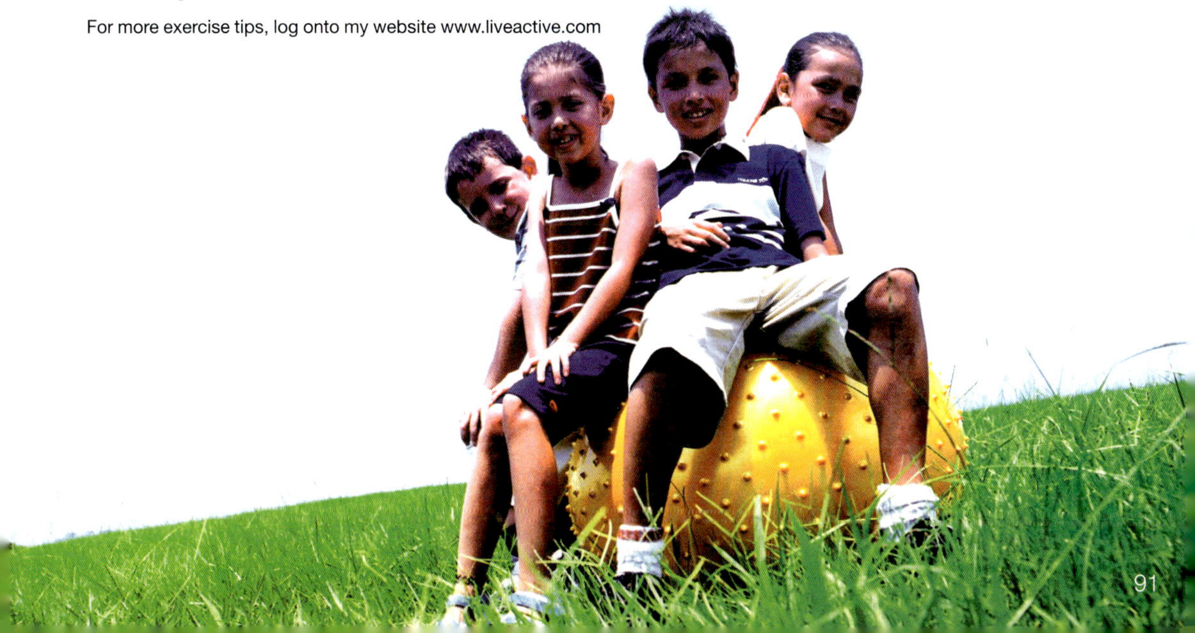

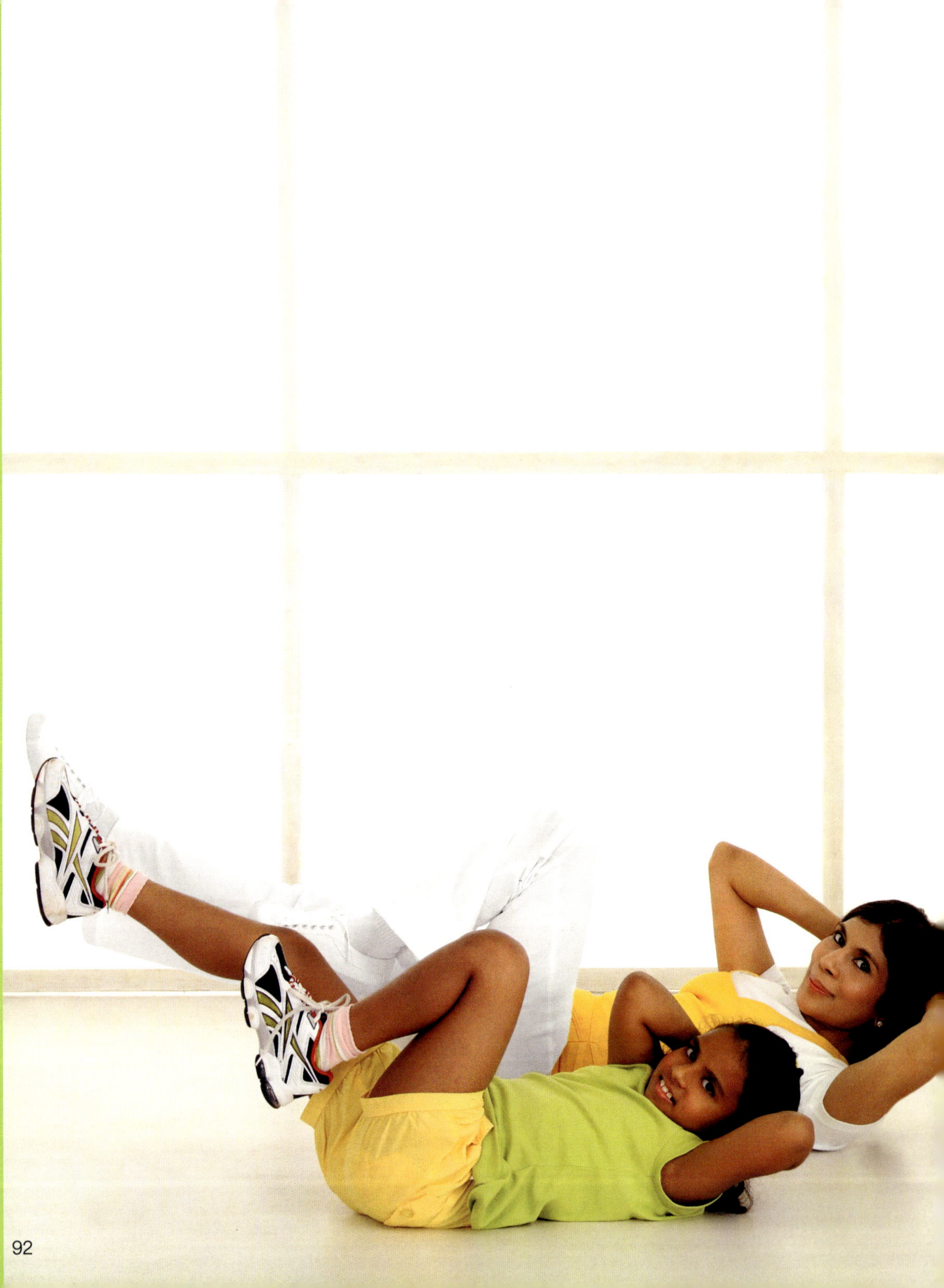

Mantra 7

Stamina. Strength. Suppleness. Stability. These are the fitness basics for raising a healthy child. Any form of **physical activity,** competitive games or free play, goes a long way in promoting fitness fundamentals.

FITTING FITNESS IN

When you watch children in a playground, you will see how active they are, jumping, running, swinging from monkey bars, cycling or performing sommersaults. Without doing it consciously, they are developing one or more of the essential fitness components - **stamina, strength, suppleness and stability – the four S's of fitness.**

stamina

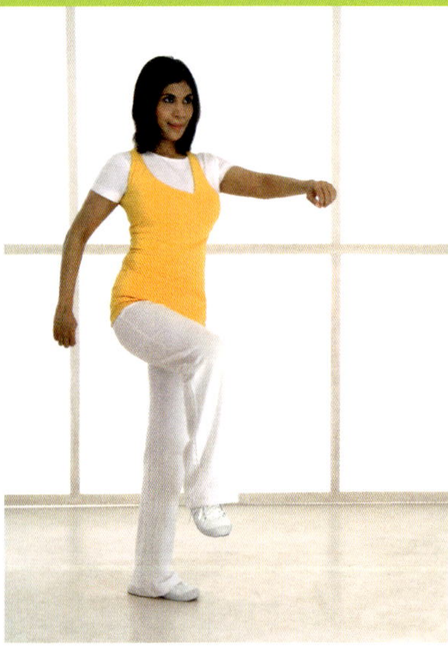

Stamina, or endurance, is developed when the body moves in a rhythmic and continuous manner, using the large muscle groups in the body. Children get this kind of exercise when they jog, run, skip, jump, or engage in sports such as swimming, cricket, tennis or squash. These exercises are essential for improving heart health. Aerobic activity gets the heart to deliver more oxygen to cells within the body.

Heart of the matter

The heart is a muscular organ located in the chest, or thoracic cavity, diagonally behind the breastbone. Similar to a clenched fist in shape and size, this small organ contracts 100,000 times a day and pumps 5 to 6 litres of blood every minute.

Q: How does exercise strengthen the heart?

A: Exercise makes the heart stronger and helps it to pump more blood with each heartbeat. A well-conditioned heart pumps more blood with fewer heartbeats, while a heart with less aerobic conditioning is not as efficient. During vigorous exercise, blood is pumped at a much quicker rate – blood can circulate upto 20 times faster than normal.

strength

Strength exercises keep your child's bones and muscles strong. When your child sits upright and walks tall, the confidence level increases. An effective strength routine would include exercises that target the major muscle groups of the upper body, mid section and lower body.

The simplest and safest way for children to improve muscle strength is to use their own body weight as resistance.

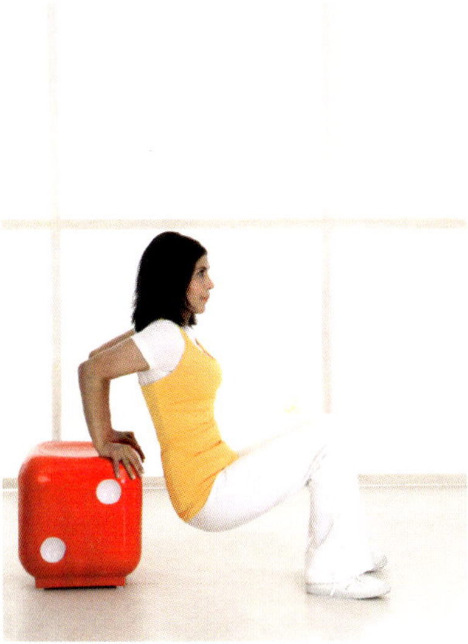

Bare bone facts

The framework of the human skeleton comprises 206 bones. Bones need calcium to grow and stay strong. Strength exercises improve calcium absorption in the bones and regular exercise actually results in increased bone density.

Myth: You have no way of knowing if your child gains strength.

FACT: Although you cannot see the body becoming stronger, you will certainly see your child demonstrate a superior performance in the level of exercise, or show increased stamina in a game. For example, when he or she plays a tennis shot, the quality of the shot will visibly improve.

Q: Will children benefit from strength training?

A: Definitely. Younger children, when supervised, will benefit from strength training exercises. They could use their body weight to execute pull-ups, push-ups and squats. Try to get your child to do the 15-minute home exercise strength routine outlined in this section.

Q: Should children lift heavy weights?

A: Children and adolescents should avoid lifting heavy weights. Power lifting and body building are also best avoided until 15 or 16 years of age. This is because any injury to the growth plate or epiphyseal plate can be risky for developing bones.

suppleness

Stretching exercises improve suppleness, allowing the body to bend and move easily through its full range of motion. These exercises promote relaxation, enhance exercise performance and keep the body agile. Even when your child bends down to tie a shoelace, the body is being stretched.

Stretching not only makes your child more flexible, it also improves posture. More specifically, the body's muscles become better coordinated. Even problems such as slouching and stooping shoulders tend to get corrected.

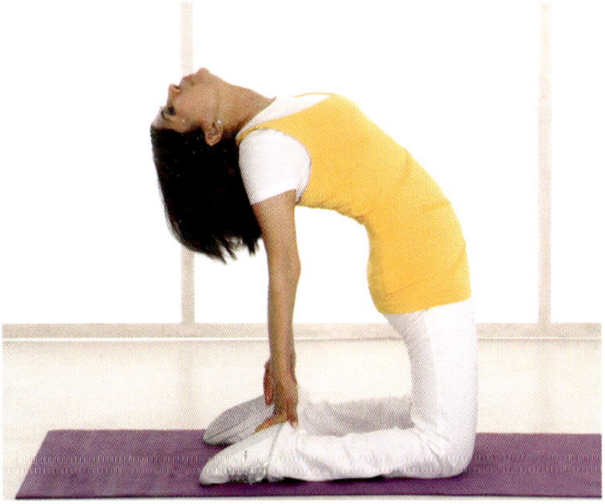

Stretch the benefits

Stretching also prevents common sports injuries. Examples are back stiffness associated with hockey, sore shoulders associated with sports like tennis, or tight leg muscles associated with running or squash. So get your child to stretch to maximum benefit.

- Stretch smoothly, never bounce.
- Breathe slowly, deeply and naturally.
- Remain relaxed and feel the stretch.

stability

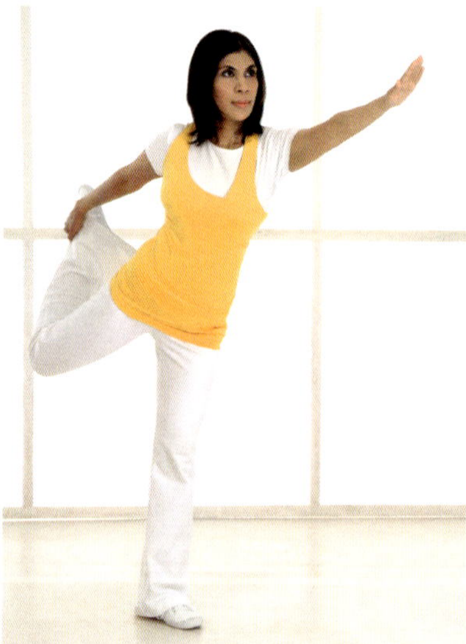

Stability, or balance training, is not something we generally think about as being part of a fitness plan. But it should be, because this activity combines reflexes, hand-eye coordination and muscle strength. When your children play games like hopscotch, turn cartwheels or skip over stones, they are using varying degrees of balance.

Benefits of balance training

- Improves functional stability for daily activities
- Improves coordination
- Enhances neuromuscular awareness
- Increases strength

Get your child to stand on one leg or on a wobble board, sit on a stability ball, roller blade, wind surf, ride a bike, inline skate or ski, to maintain and improve the inherent balancing abilities.

FIT Fact

Sports of all types require a sense of balance, whether it is clearing a hurdle or reaching out to catch a ball.

begin with a warm-up

To prevent injury, it is important for your child to warm up before exercising. Just as a car revvs up into first gear and starts moving, the body too gets into gear with a warm-up.

A warm-up gradually elevates the heart rate and boosts circulation. It primes the cardio-respiratory system and musculoskeletal system to prepare for the exercises that will follow. Remind your child to start gradually and build up the intensity in time.

A warm-up should include about 5 minutes of light activity, such as walking, spot-marching, knee lifts, jogging and stretching.

end with a cool-down

It is also important for your child to cool down after exercising. Stopping exercise abruptly, without a cool-down period, can result in a rapid drop in blood pressure. Your child may also suffer from cramps and lightheadedness. Like the warm-up, 5 minutes of light activity is required to cool down.

The cool-down helps your child's heart rate to gradually return to normal. It also helps to eliminate toxic waste, such as lactic acid, that builds up in the muscles.

TWO WAYS TO GET YOUR CHILD TO COOL DOWN

- Continue chosen exercise while gradually slowing its intensity (especially if it is a high intensity activity). Gradually slowing down the pace and exertion of the activity, over a 5-10 minute period, is a natural cool-down process.
- Stretch to cool down. Just after high-energy exercise, the muscles are still warm and, as they are stretched, they relax. Stretching is also great for improving suppleness.

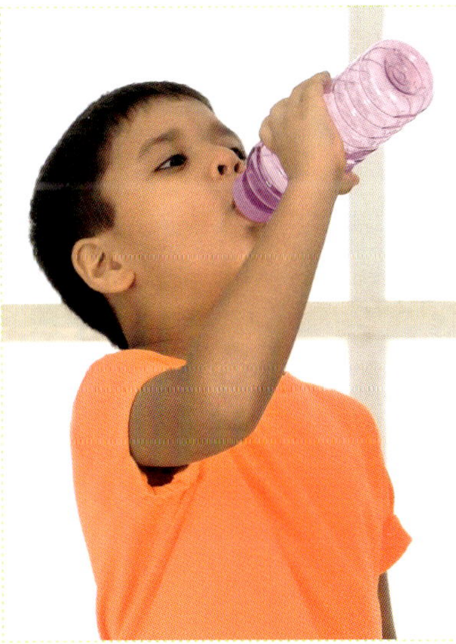

Q: Is your child water starved?

A: Make sure your child drinks plenty of water before, after, and during an exercise routine. Schedule water breaks during play to prevent heatstroke, dizziness and dehydration. Particularly after play, your child must drink water to keep the body cool and replace lost fluids.

Thirst is not the only indicator of how much fluid your child has lost and is therefore not an accurate method of determining how much water your child needs to consume. It is therefore important to ensure your child continues drinking water to stay hydrated.

PRE-WORKOUT CHECKLIST

- Always start with a warm-up as part of the workout session.
- Wear comfortable clothing and shoes that offer adequate support.
- Drink plenty of water before starting to exercise.
- After a meal, allow for a 90-minute gap before exercise.

POST-WORKOUT CHECKLIST

- Include a cool-down after exercise.
- Drink plenty of water.
- Give your child a fruit shake or a nutritious snack if hungry.

EASE YOUR CHILD INTO THE ROUTINE, GRADUALLY

- Exercising too much, too soon, too quickly, are the main causes of injuries. Make sure your child's exercise program is systematic and progressive.
- Focus on right form and technique, to protect the joints.
- Rest is important, as it helps the muscles to get rid of exhaustion and recuperate from the stress of exercise.

the 15-minute home strength routine

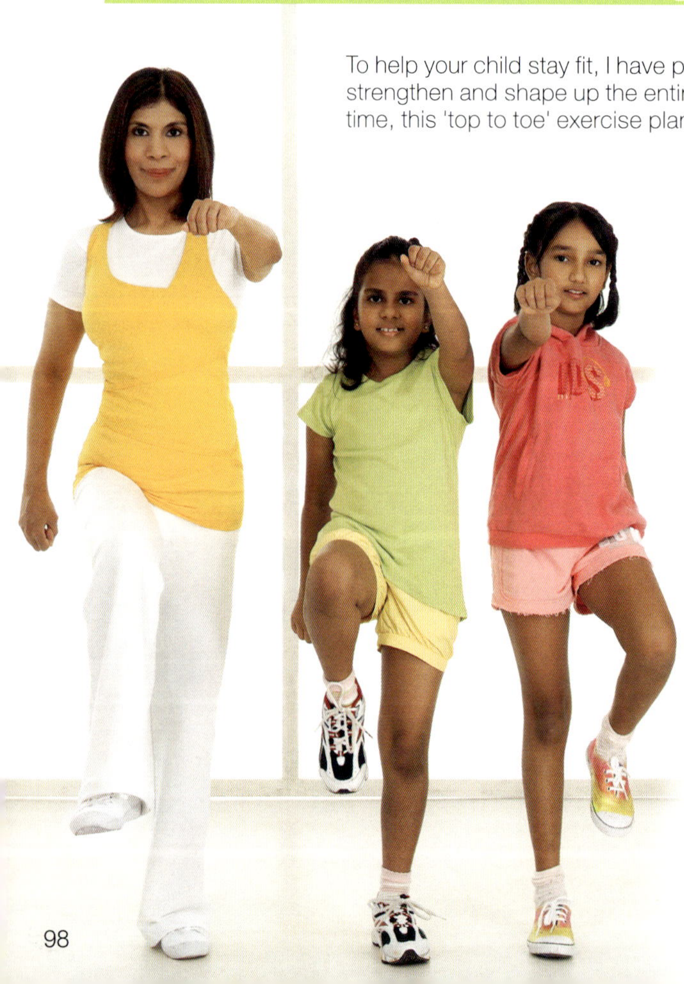

To help your child stay fit, I have put together a total body workout plan to strengthen and shape up the entire body. In just 15 minutes of available time, this 'top to toe' exercise plan will have your child fighting fit!

- calf raise
- squats
- lunge
- tricep dip
- push-ups
- abdominal crunch
- oblique bicycle
- alternate arm & leg raise

The step-by-step instructions that follow are for your child. The exercises can be done thrice a week on alternate days.

Start with a brisk 5-minute walk to warm-up.

calf raise

repeat 16 counts
benefit shapes and strengthens calf muscles
target gastrocnemius & soleus muscles

This is one of the most effective exercises to strengthen and tone the calves.

1. Stand tall, with shoulders back and chest lifted.
2. Come up on your toes and, balancing on the balls of your feet, lift your heels as high as possible. Slowly, lower your heels. Breathe out as you lift, breathe in as you lower.

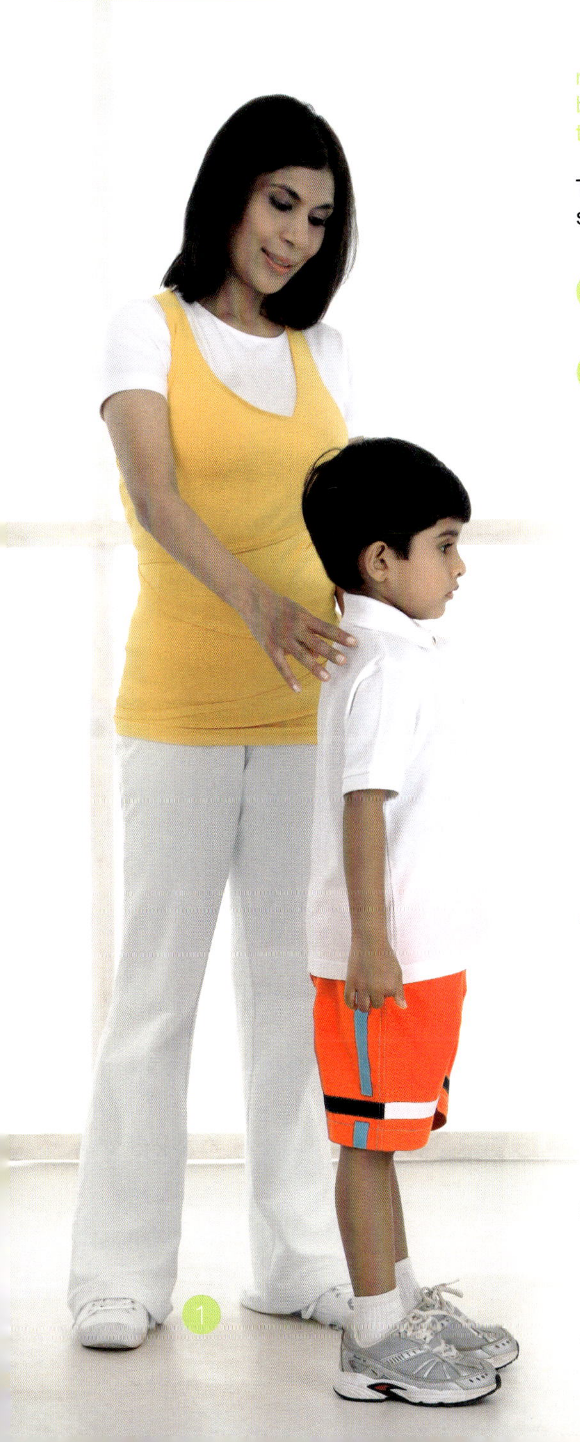

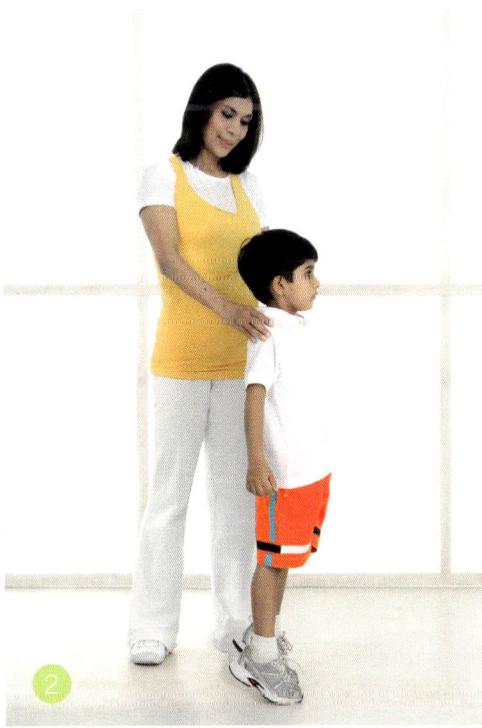

squats

repeat 16 counts
benefit strengthens the hips and thighs
target gluteus maximus, hamstrings and quadricep muscles

This is an excellent move to shape the hips and thighs. To avoid straining the knees do not jerk up from the squat position, especially while extending your legs.

1. Stand tall, keeping your feet hip-width apart.
2. Bend your knees to about a 90-degree angle and lower into a squat position. Make sure your knees do not go over your toes. Return to starting position.

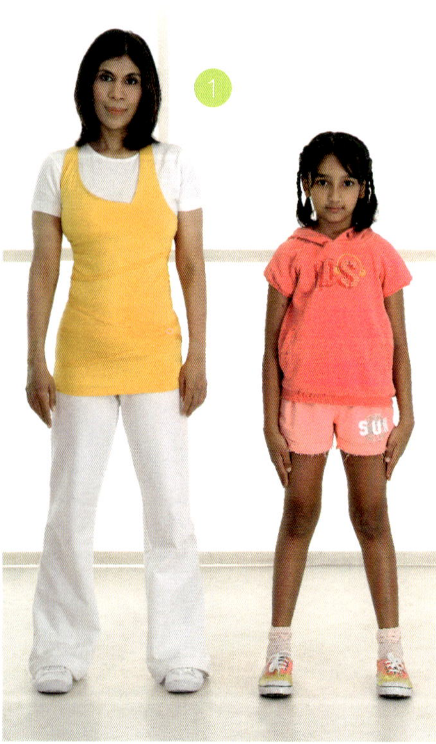

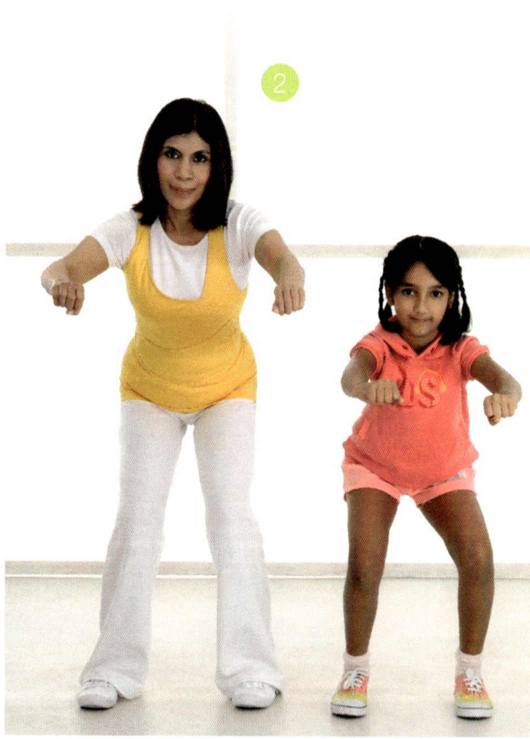

lunge

repeat 16 counts
benefit strengthens the hips and thighs
target gluteus maximus, hamstrings and quadricep muscles

This exercise targets the muscles of the lower body, giving them a firmer and more sculpted appearance. Hold your abs in and keep your feet planted firmly on the floor while performing this exercise.

1. Stand with your feet hip-width apart and bring one foot forward.
2. Bend your knees and lower into a lunge position. Make sure your knees are in line with your ankles or toes. Return to start position and switch legs.

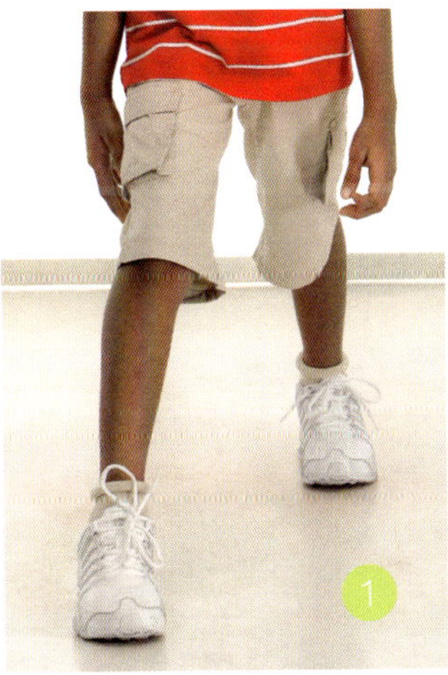

1

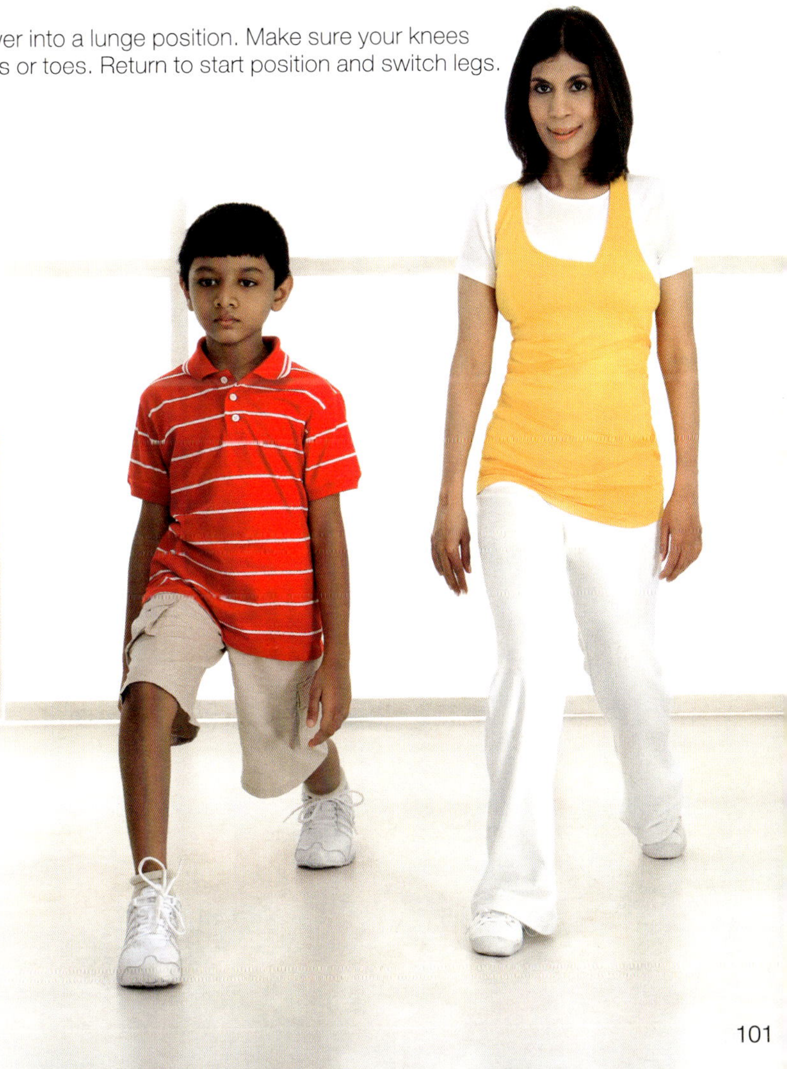

2

tricep dip

repeat 16 counts
benefit tones and sculpts triceps
target tricep muscles

This upper arm exercise works the back of the arms. These muscles need to be strengthened as they are usually not as strong as the front of the arm.

1. With your back to a stool or chair, position your legs in front of you, keeping your knees bent.
2. Grip the edge of the stool and bend your arms so that you descend towards the floor. Use your triceps to push back up to starting position.

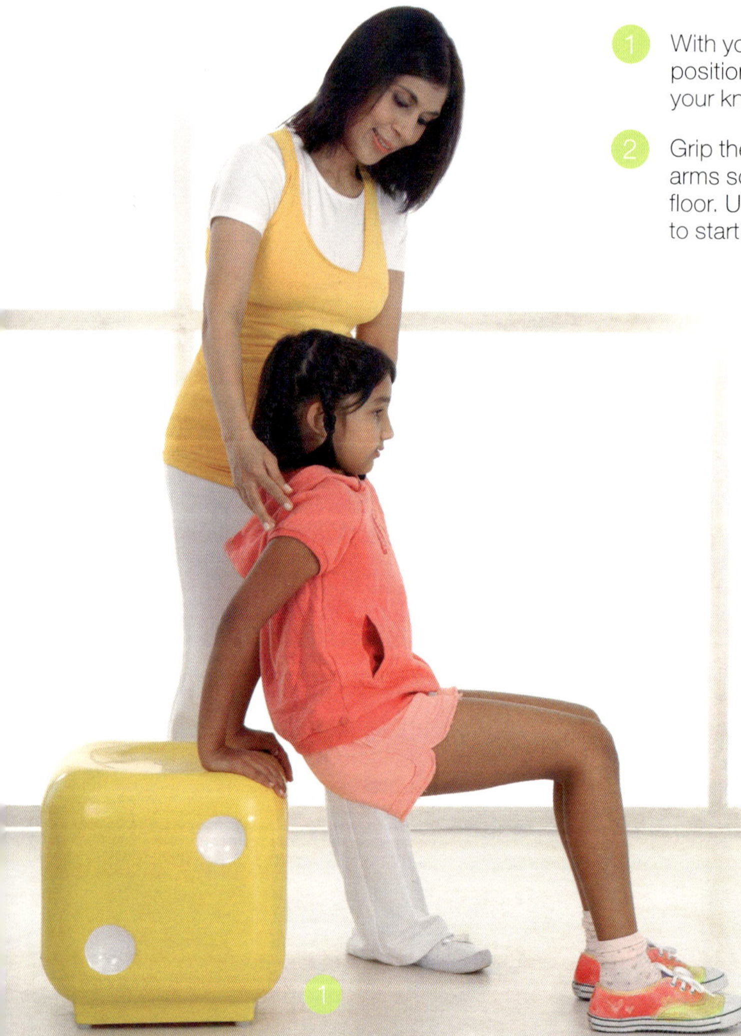

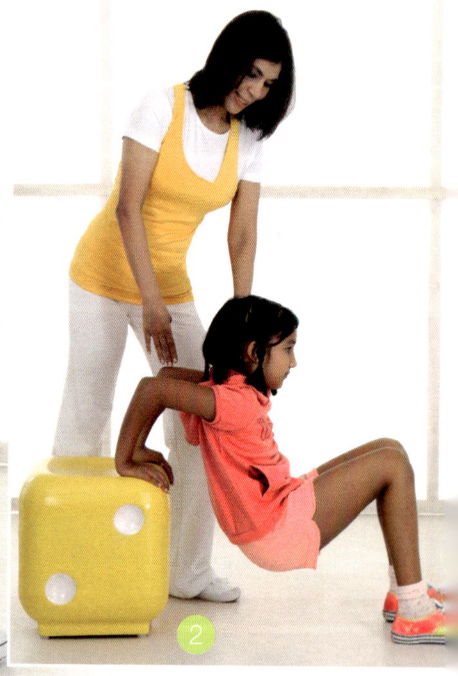

push-ups

repeat 16 counts
benefit strengthens upper body
target pectorals, triceps, deltoids

This exercise primarily targets the large muscles of the upper body – the chest, triceps and shoulders.

1. Place your hands directly under your shoulders and keep your fingers pointing forwards, toes planted on the ground and your back straight.

2. Slowly bend your elbows and lower your body, bringing your chest close to the floor, and then return to starting position.

1

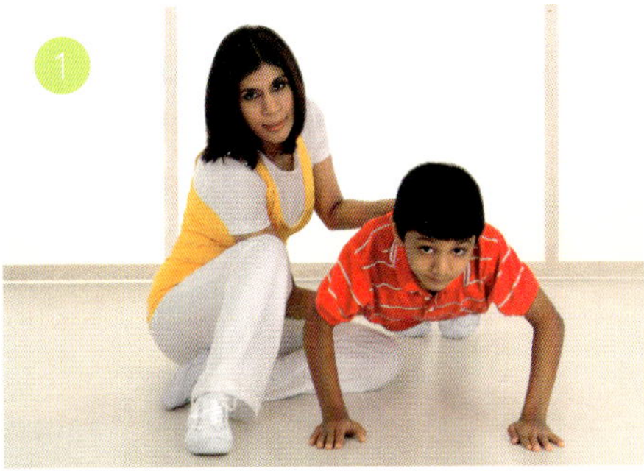

2

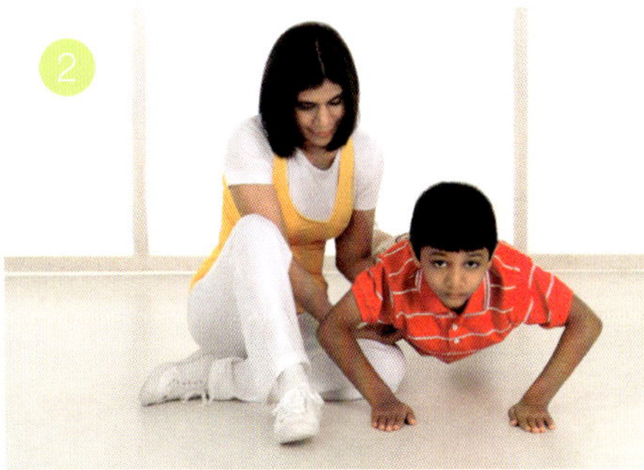

abs crunch

repeat 16 counts
benefit tones and tightens abdominal muscles
target rectus abdominis muscle

1. Lie on your back with your hands placed behind your head. Bend knees, with feet shoulder-width apart.

2. Raise legs and bend the knees to a 90 angle. Now raise your shoulders slowly, feel the abdominal muscles contract. Slowly lower down. Breathe out as you lift, breathe in as you lower.

1

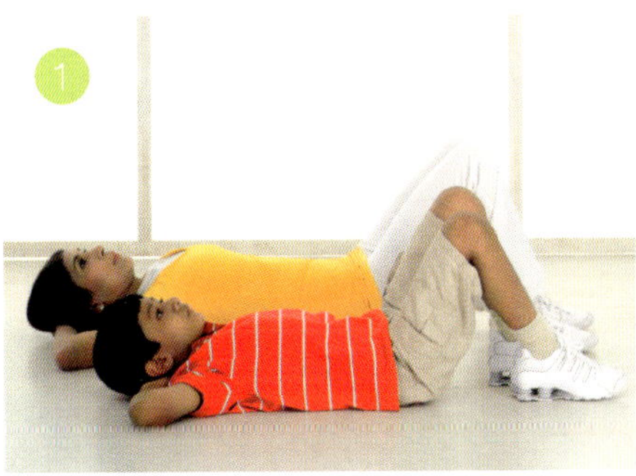

2

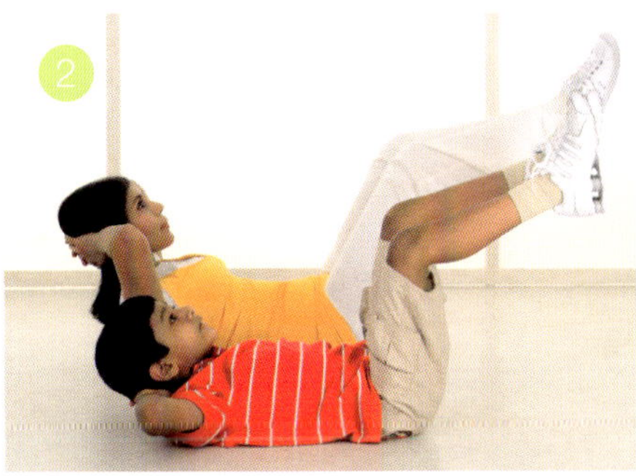

oblique bicycle

repeat 16 counts
benefit works the waist muscles
target oblique muscles

Aim to get the shoulder as close as possible to your knee. The closer you get, the better it is for your waist.

1. Lie on your back with legs bent and arms behind your head to support your neck.

2. Keeping your chin off the chest, slowly contract your abs and bring your right elbow toward your left knee, twisting to the left side, then bring your left elbow toward your right knee twisting to the right side.

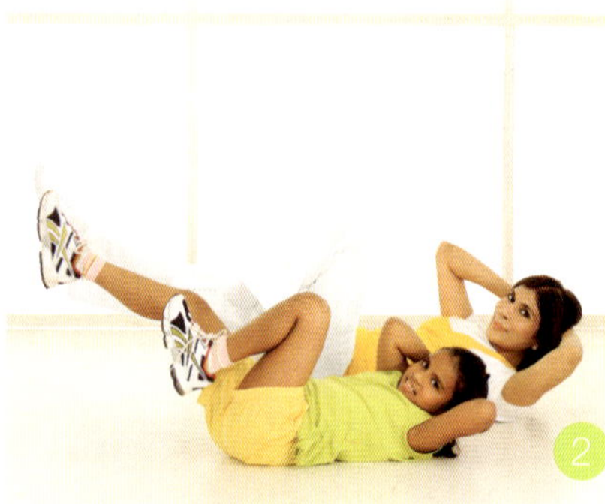

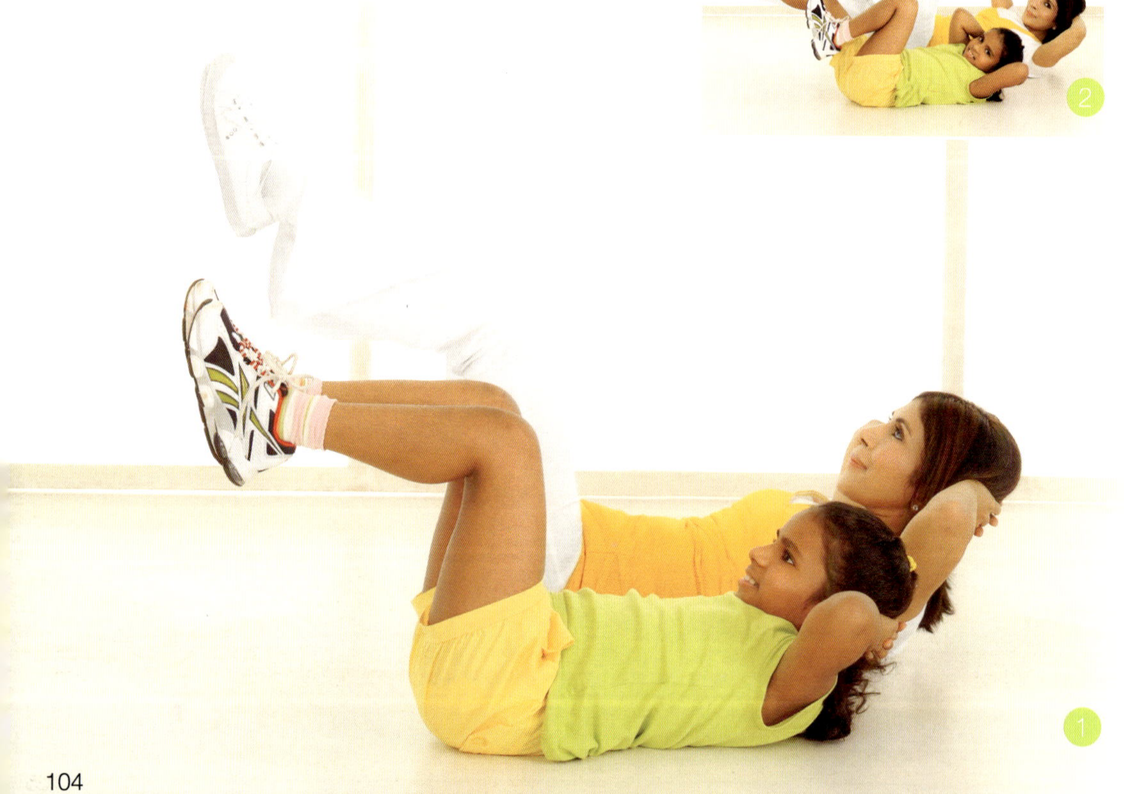

alternate arm & leg raise

repeat 16 counts
benefit strengthens the diagonal back muscles
target gluteus maximus, errector spinae, posterior deltoid

This exercise resembles Superman in the prone position! While lifting, stretch your legs and arms out, and make sure your neck is relaxed and in line with your spine.

1. Lie on your stomach on the mat.

2. Raise your left arm and right leg, keeping them straight. Lower the arm and leg. Now, raise your right arm and left leg. Lower.

2

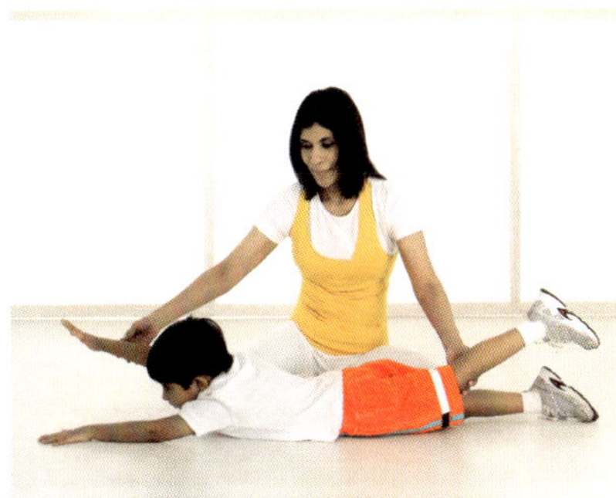

1

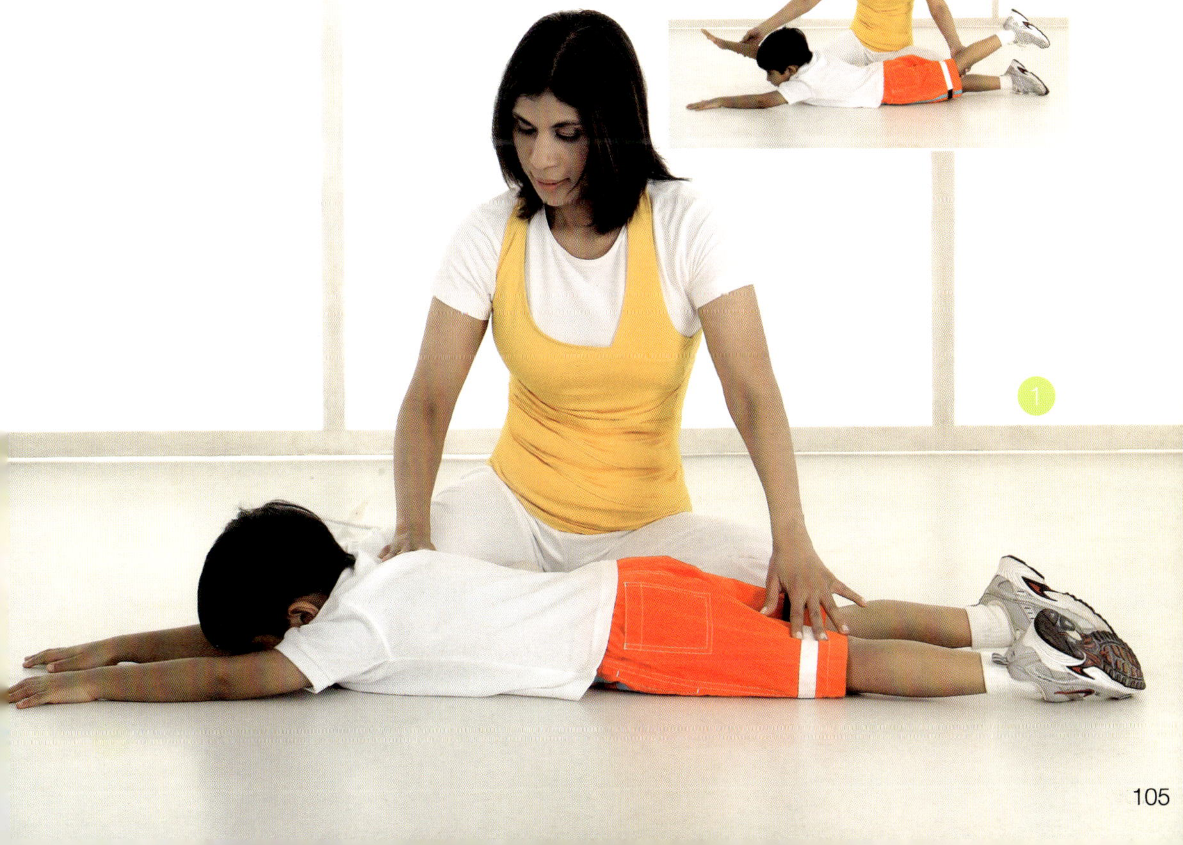

stretches

Stretching has so many benefits, you can actually feel the results immediately! When muscles in the body are tense or overworked, stretching releases the stiffness. In the long term, stretching improves posture and flexibility, and enhances muscle coordination. It is one of the key components of a balanced fitness programme.

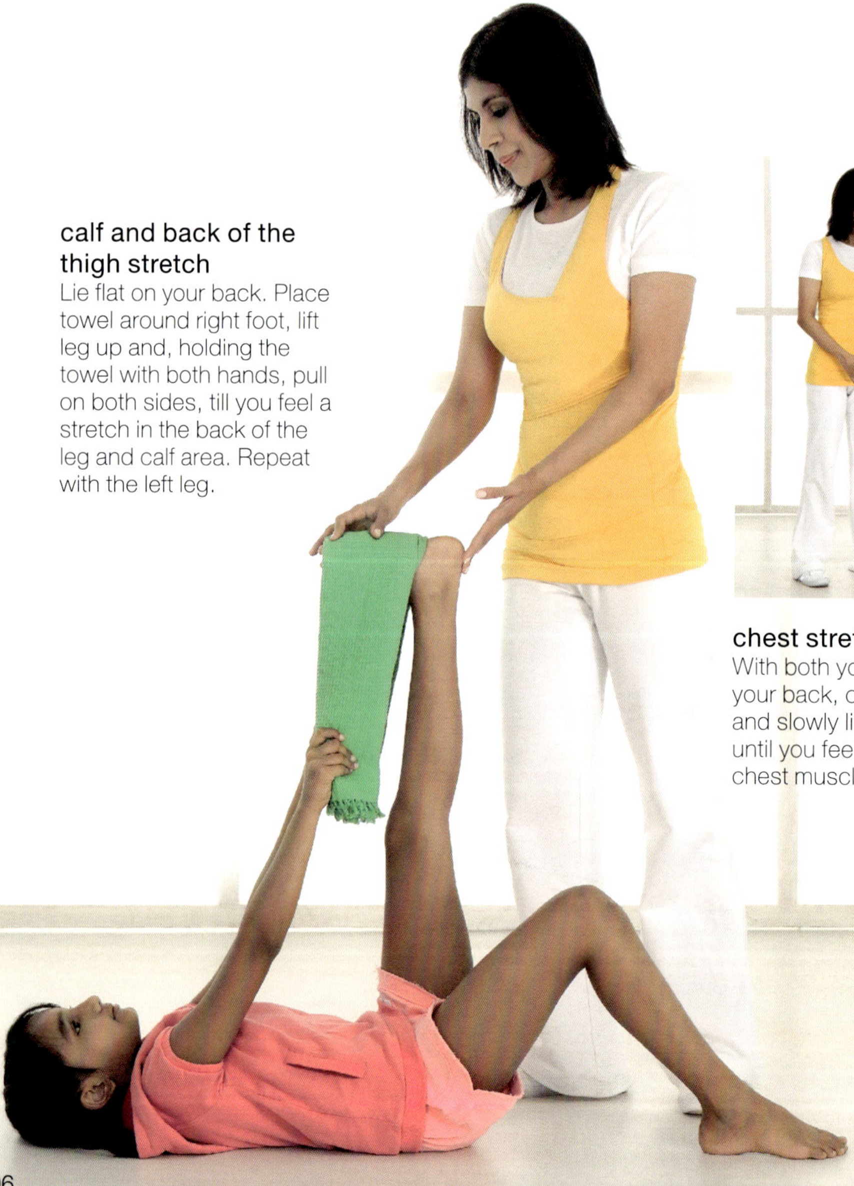

calf and back of the thigh stretch

Lie flat on your back. Place towel around right foot, lift leg up and, holding the towel with both hands, pull on both sides, till you feel a stretch in the back of the leg and calf area. Repeat with the left leg.

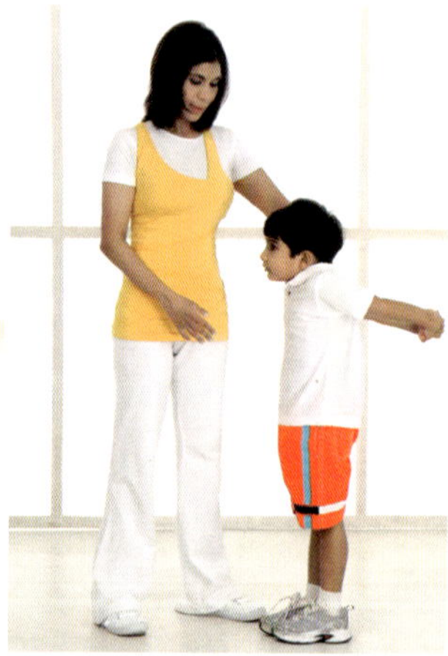

chest stretch

With both your hands behind your back, clasp your fingers and slowly lift your hands up until you feel a stretch in your chest muscles and pectorals.

shoulder rolls

Rotate your shoulders forward 5 times and then in reverse direction 5 times.

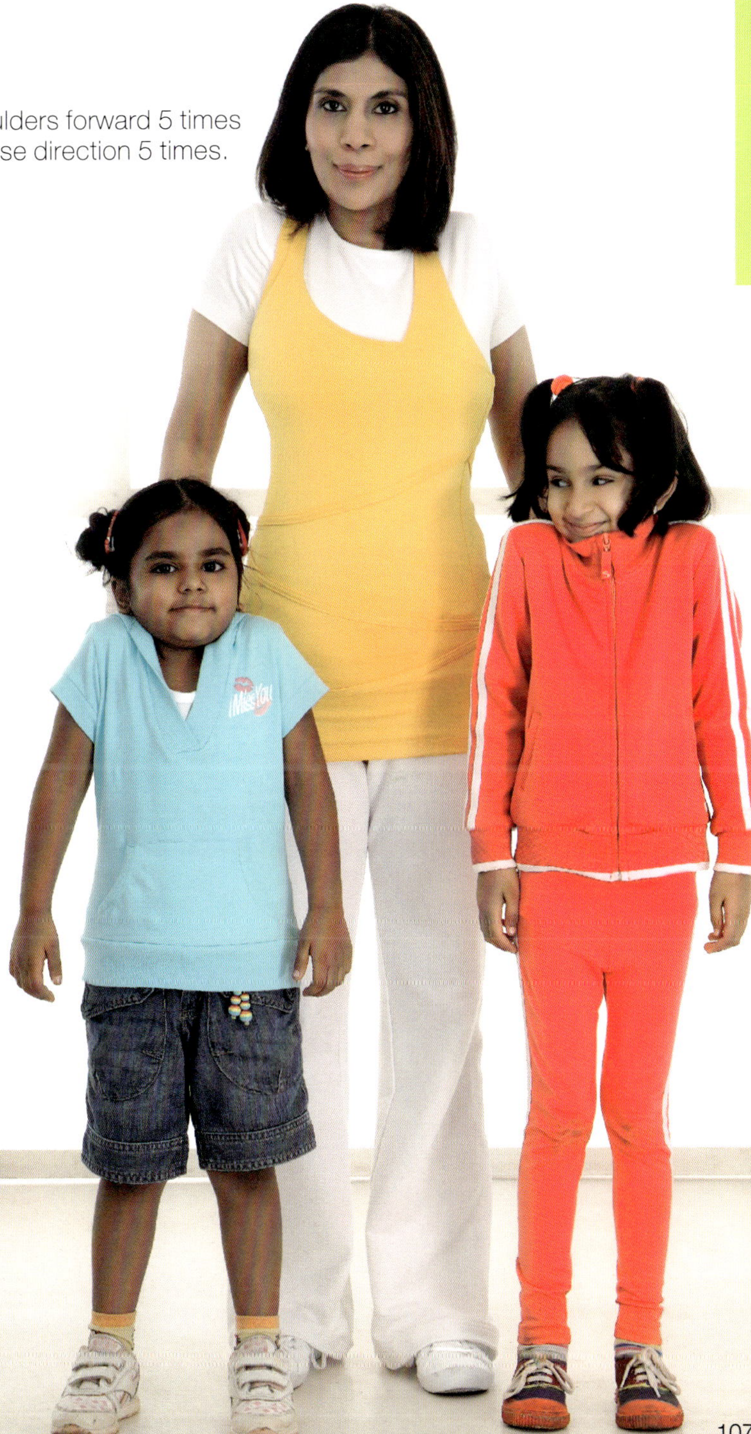

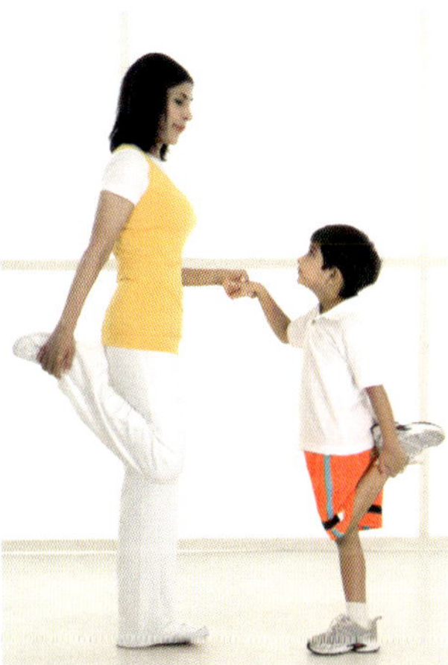

front of the thigh stretch

Stand tall. Grasp right foot with right hand. Bring your foot toward buttocks, keeping knees together. Hold and repeat with the other leg.

HOLD It!

- Hold each stretch for 10 to 30 seconds.
- Do not hold your breath when you stretch!

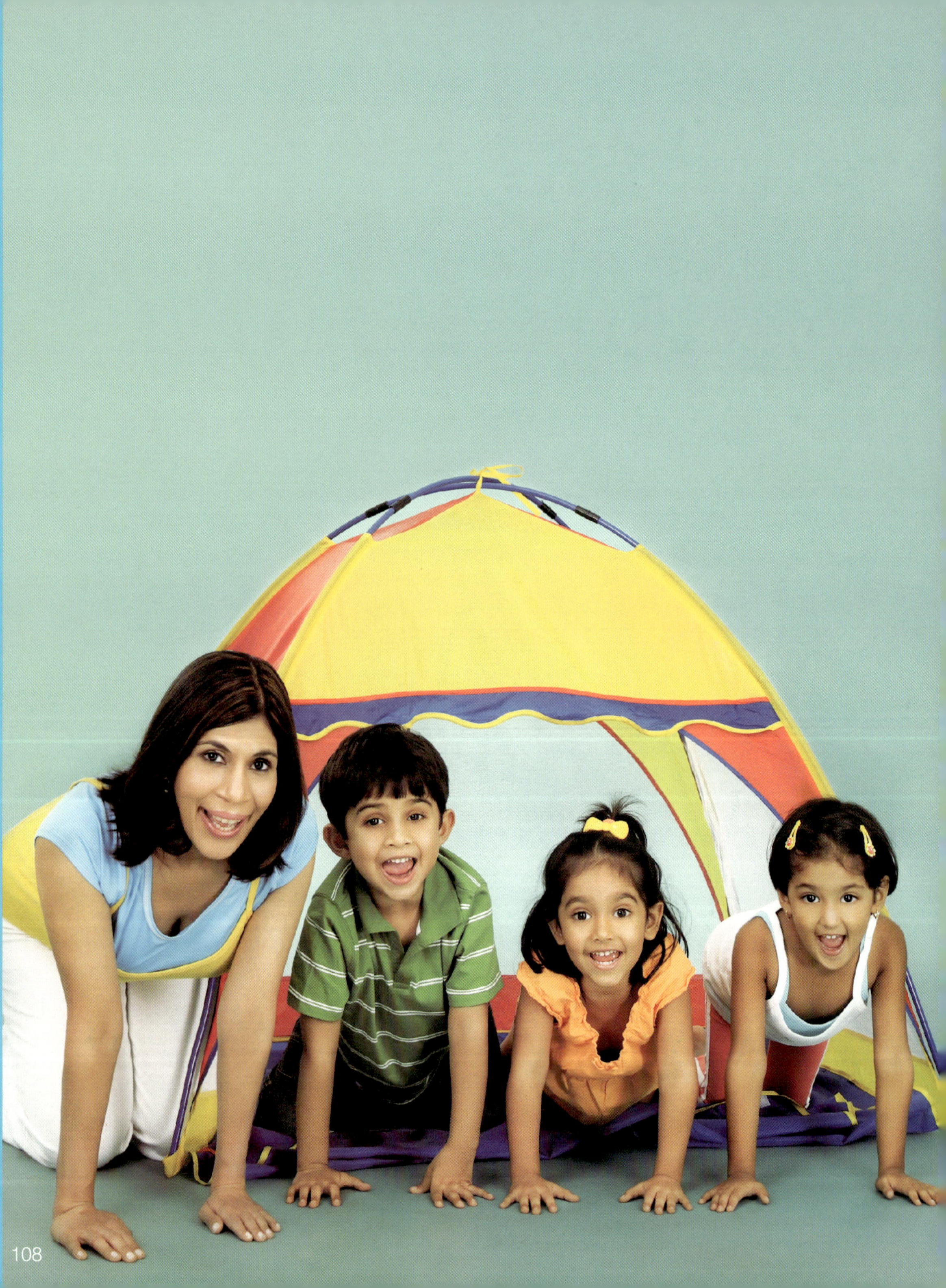

Mantra 8

Got 5 minutes? Time need not be a constraint for **physical activity.** Even **5 minutes** of exercise helps to ward off lethargy and boredom - see how much your child can accomplish within a **limited time** span.

HOMEACTIVE: GOT 5 MINUTES?

5 minutes every day sets fitness habits for a lifetime. Believe it or not, even a small pocket of time, as little as 5 minutes, makes a difference in raising a healthier child. It's not hard to do. Children are, by nature, physically active. They enjoy any form of hopping, skipping, running, climbing, or showing off their skills with a ball. So if you have some interesting suggestions to offer, your children are sure to jump at the opportunity!

The next time your kids say, "I'm bored", you know exactly what to do. Introduce a fun physical activity that they will really enjoy. Think back to the time you were a child... Moms, did you play hopscotch? Dads, did you play gully cricket with your building buddies?

Of course, kids today are different. Get your kids to try out a range of different activities, to figure what they consider "fun". Keep in mind, if activities become too regimented, or too rule-driven, children will run a mile before they think of getting involved!

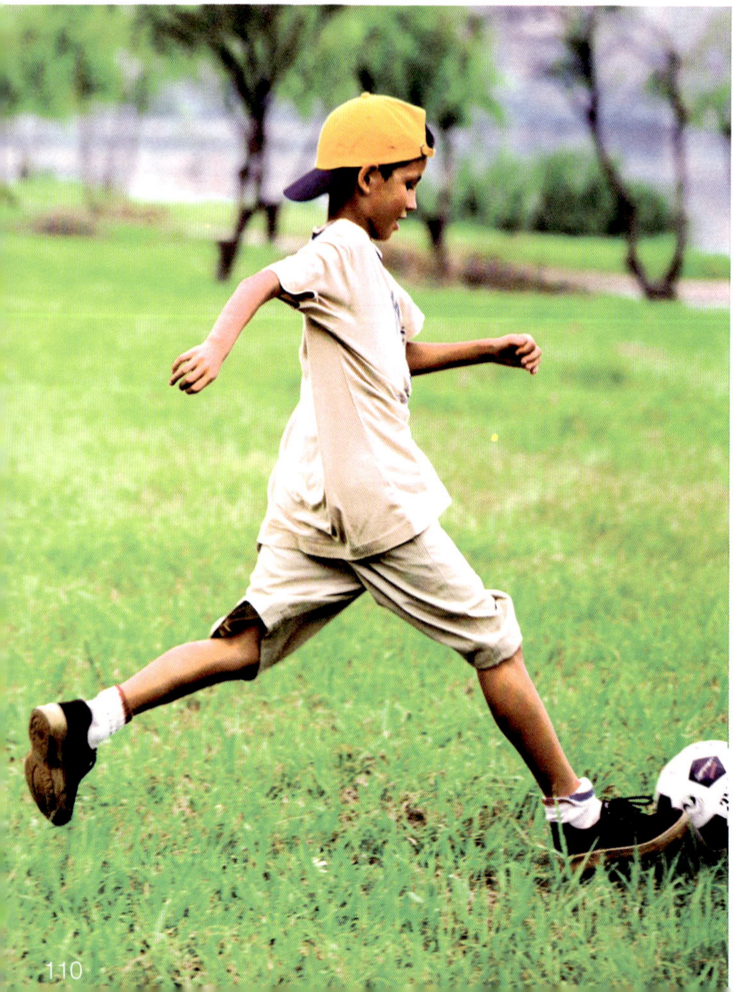

Fitness does not have to come with a price tag. Whether your kids prefer running, cycling, skipping or even dribbling a ball, it doesn't matter, as long as they are active.

The important thing is to remind your children, every day, that they must get out of the house to play. You could buy them some basic equipment – a bat and ball, a skipping rope, or skates. You will be surprised how creative kids can be even with simple resources. They use their imaginations to role play, set up teams, or invent some new game. Often, they don't even need any equipment, just chasing one another around the building is a form of sport.

The best part is, kids lose track of time when they are happily engaged in an activity they enjoy. Buddy activities can keep children going for hours on end. They are so busy having a good time, that they seldom stop to think how much effort they are putting in towards being fit.

I have listed here, from 1 to 10, activities that kids enjoy. Some are for smaller children, while most are ideal for kids of all ages. Check what your child might want to pick up.

1. imitate animals or birds (such as froggy jump, birds flapping wings)
2. skipping
3. cycling
4. play with a ball (basket ball, dribble, or wall ball)
5. jump on the trampoline
6. use the hula hoop
7. hurdle jump
8. play with a Frisbee or play phoogadi
9. skating
10. hopscotch

1 imitate animals

Put your small child's love for imitating to good use. Try to get him or her to do the frog jump, flap wings like a bird, or stand on one leg like a stork. Kids also love galloping like horses, swinging like monkeys on a monkey bar, or even something as simple as stretching out like a cat.

BENEFITS: Encourages creativity, while the movements increase strength and stamina.

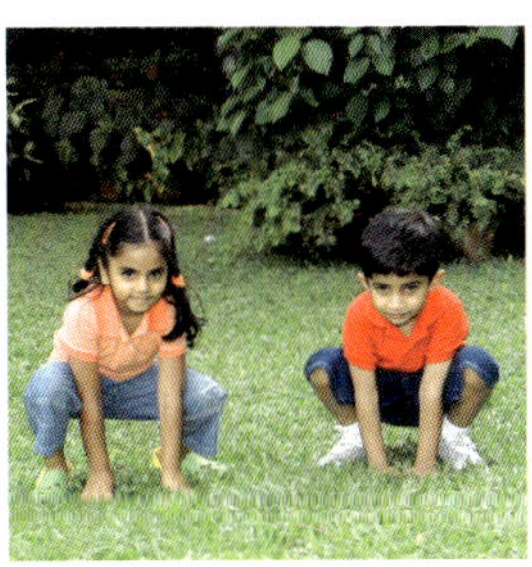
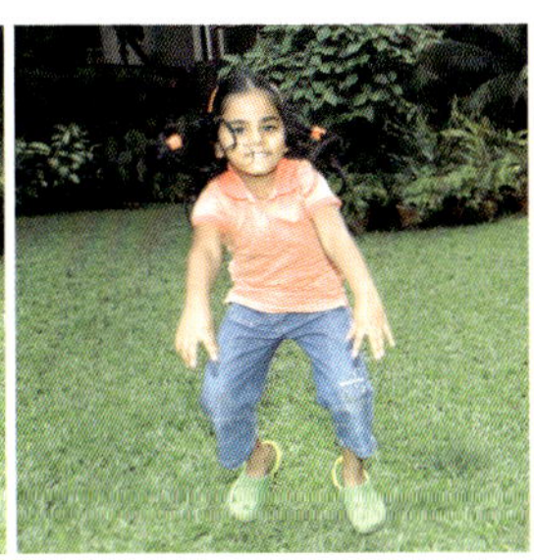
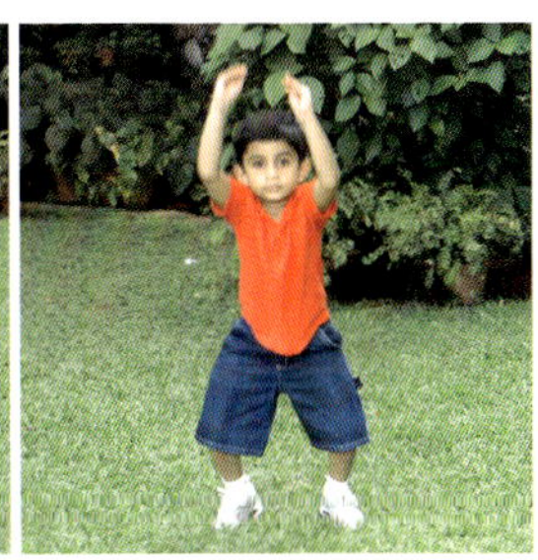

2 skipping

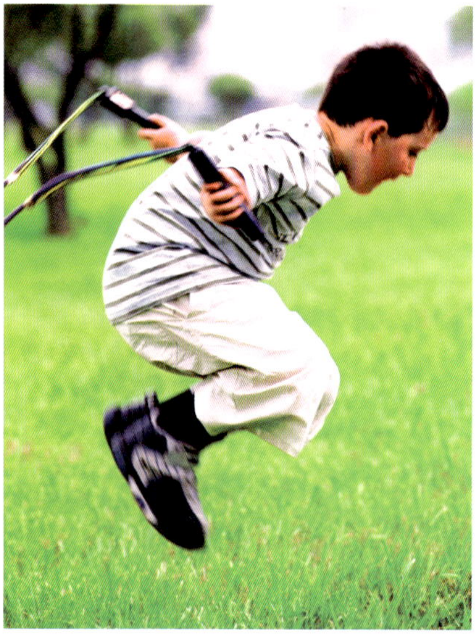

Skipping is convenient and does not require a lot of space or any special equipment. A skipping rope is something you can carry anywhere. Rope jumping improves with practice. Soon your child will develop rhythmic movements for the arms and legs, as the body moves in synchrony with the skipping rope.

ROPE LENGTH: To determine the correct length of rope, get your child to place the centre of the rope under one foot. Make him stand up straight. Then, holding the ends of the rope, get him to bring his arms to his sides, in line with the shoulders, with the rope gripped completely taut. This length of rope is right for the user.

If you have two kids, of almost the same height, they could share a skipping rope, but if there is a big height difference, it is better to get two separate ropes, one for each.

WHY SKIP?

With its circular rhythmic movement, skipping strengthens the muscles of the legs and arms. It is an excellent exercise for the heart and lungs, and is considered one of the most efficient workouts to increase cardiovascular fitness.

3 cycling

Cycling is considered a low-impact aerobic activity. This form of exercise does not put any stress on the knee joints, because the cyclist's weight rests on the bicycle seat.

Cycling indoors or outdoors can be an exciting experience! Outdoor cycling along park trails, beaches or around the neighbourhood is great exercise. For children, cycling on roads must be strictly supervised. It is important they know the rules of the road before they get out.

Indoor cycling is fun too. Your kids could join "spin" or other cycle classes, with some of their friends. If you live in a high-traffic city, this is a safe way to get the benefit of cycling, without having to step outdoors.

BENEFITS: Cycling is beneficial for toning the legs and like any form of regular aerobic exercise, cycling enhances energy levels and reduces stress.

TECHNIQUE: Good posture is very important when cycling. Make sure your child makes the necessary adjustments to the bicycle to keep posture correct. The following points must be kept in mind, whether cycling indoors on a machine, or outdoors.

- Keep the ball and front of your foot placed firmly on the pedals.
- Maintain good posture at all times, as there may be a tendency to hunch over the handlebars when your child is tired.
- Ensure that the cycle is the correct size for your child's height and limb length.
- Adjust seat height. At the lowest part of the cycle action, the leg should be slightly bent. If your child has to straighten out the leg completely, it means the seat is too high. This puts unnecessary strain on the knee joint.

4 basket ball, dribble, or wall ball

Any activity that involves playing with a ball improves hand-eye coordination. When your child plays football or any racquet sport, coordinated reflexes and the ability to strategize are match winners. It takes hours of daily practice, dribbling, throwing, catching, passing, to achieve a certain level of proficiency in any sport.

Younger kids just need to familiarize themselves with playing ball. The little ones can play "catch catch", throwing the ball back and forth to each other. If they are by themselves, wall ball is the perfect option. Just get a small rubber ball that they can bounce against a wall, and then catch.

There is a little rhyme that has been used by kids, for years, to play wall ball.

OLIVER TWIST	One wall bounce
CAN YOU DO THIS	One wall bounce
IF SO	Two wall bounces
DO SO	Two wall bounces
TOUCH YOUR KNEES	One wall bounce and touching knees
TOUCH YOUR TOES	One wall bounce and touching toes
BOUNCE THE BALL	One floor bounce
UNDER YOU GO	Lift leg, throw ball from under the leg, one wall bounce

5 trampoline

Your kids can bounce their way to a fitter body. Trampoline rebounding is a great way to lose weight, gain cardiovascular benefits and have fun, while working out at the same time.

TRAMPOLINE BASICS: Gymnasts and acrobats often use an elevated elastic canvas or net bed as a performing surface. The trampoline is a little more than just that. A spring or rubber suspension anchors the elastic canvas bed and the springs beneath lift the body with an upward bounce.

ON THE REBOUND: Rebounding is unique since it uses the natural laws of gravity to stimulate every cell of the body. We are all subject to gravity, but on the trampoline, the body moves against gravity.

IS IT SAFE?

Yes, rebounding on the trampoline is safe and cushions the impact on the joints. For example, when you run, or exercise on a solid surface, a certain amount of force from the impact is felt in the body. On the trampoline, it is a bit like "swimming" on air, because the mat absorbs the impact, almost like an air bubble, breaking your kids' fall as they come down.

Apart from the physics of defying gravity, kids simply love the idea of jumping higher and higher, with the trampoline giving them more height each time they jump.

6 hula hoop

Hula hooping is a fun game that you might have played as a kid. It involves rotating the waist rapidly, to keep a large hoop circling around the waist in midair. This is a great belly and waist move – belly dancers were probably inspired by the hula hoop!

The hula hoop gives your child a great body workout, particularly around the torso. Coordination of body movements strengthens torso muscles and enhances flexibility of the spine.

Children enjoy keeping the hula hoop going, often competing in time to see who can set a record! Hula hoops are available in metal and plastic versions at sports stores.

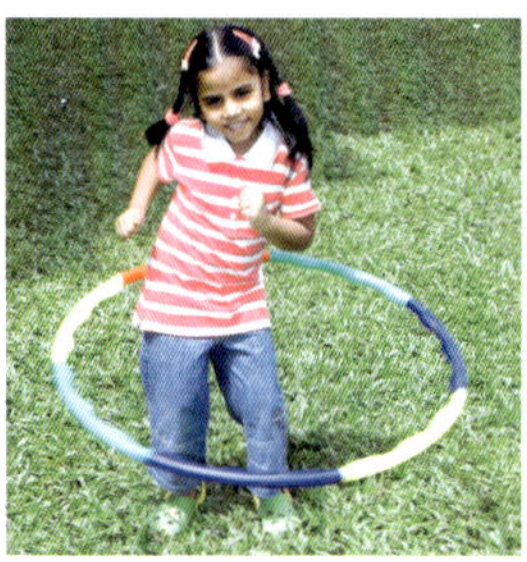
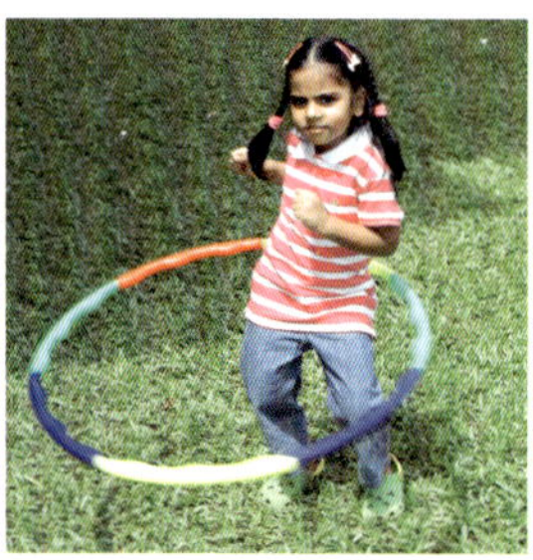
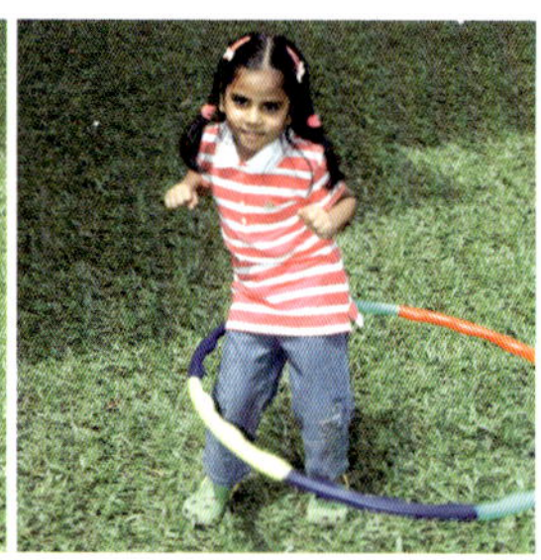

7 skating

Skating is a great skill for children of all ages. Kids have a natural sense of balance, and this can be developed in the early years. Once they get their balance, children love the freedom of gliding around on wheels.

Skating is a fun way to stay fit - get the children out in the building compound, but make sure they avoid main roads, unless they stick to the pavement.

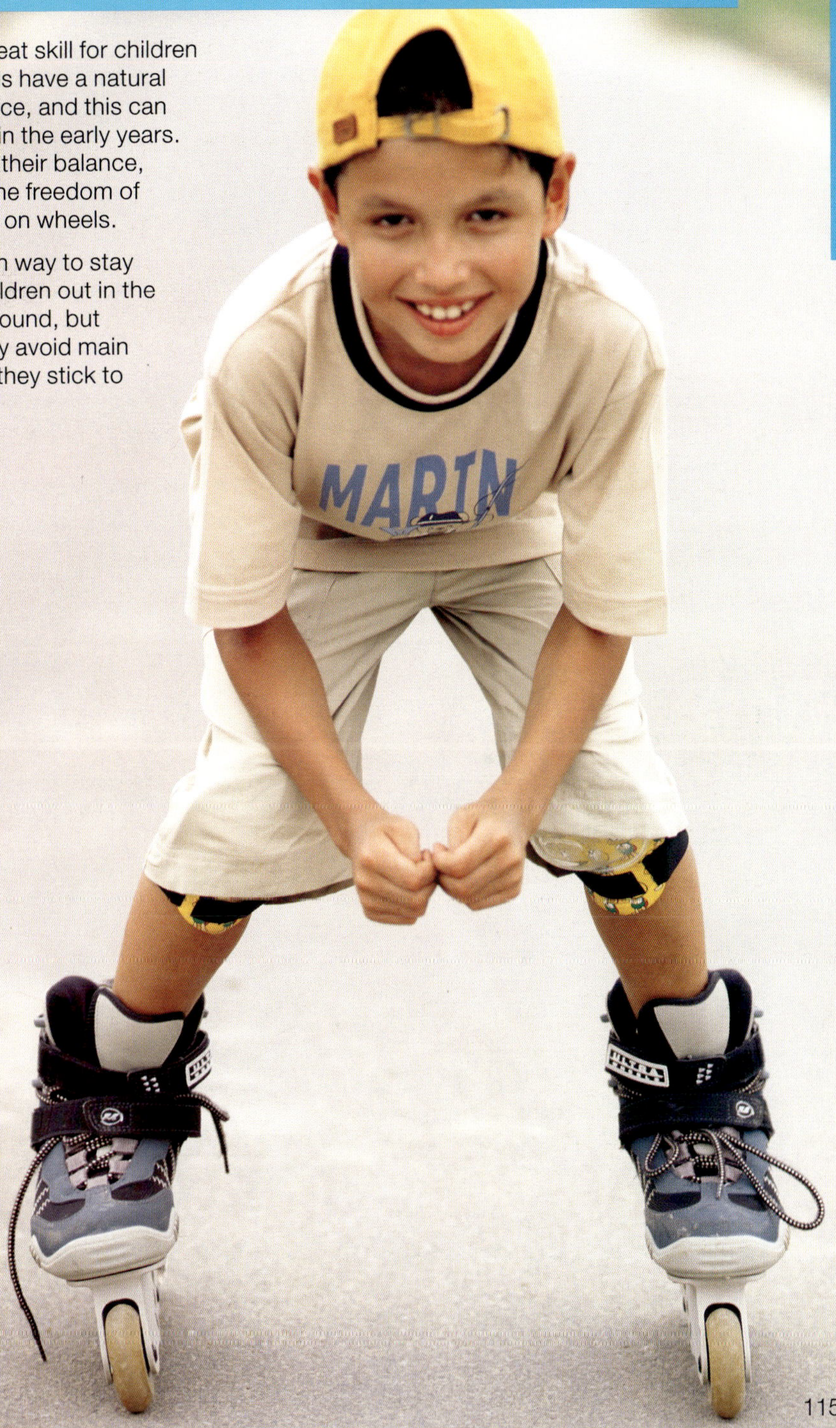

8 hurdle jump

As you know, the hurdle jump is included as an Olympic event. This activity requires a high degree of fitness, strength and stamina.

Hurdle jumps involve controlled jumps, leaps and bounds. When an athlete jumps, the body must be able to flex and extend quickly, to get propelled upwards with the maximum force.

Your child will be doing hurdles at a basic level. Make sure kids warm up slightly before hurdle jumping, so they are ready for this high impact activity.

Competitive kids tend to enjoy hurdle jumping. They see it as a challenge. Initially, your little ones can start by jumping over cushions and small objects. Once they master this, they will want to jump over more challenging targets!

At the school level, your older child may want to continue to participate in long jump, high jump, or hurdles. Encourage them to set personal goals that they can achieve.

9 playing with a Frisbee

When your child just wants to try something a little different, instead of playing ball as a regular past-time, introduce the Frisbee. Available in colourful discs, Frisbees look like flying saucers soaring up in the sky. The throwing technique also differs from a ball and requires good judgment.

The interesting part is, Frisbees tend to pick up air currents, and are therefore unpredictable. If your child throws it in one direction, the Frisbee can take off in another! This delights children, who are happy to run about trying to catch it.

This is a stress-free pursuit, just the thing your child needs to unwind, especially after long hours of sitting in school.

10 hopscotch

A fun game where you twist, turn, jump and hop! Hopscotch requires a minimum of 2 players and can involve up to 4. Each player gets their turn to throw a flat stone into the hopscotch squares, and hop from square to square.

- Mark out the hopscotch square as shown in the picture on right.
- A player starts by throwing the stone into square 1. If the stone falls within the square, the player hops all the way up on the single squares and places both legs down on the double squares, till numbers 7 and 8. The player then returns by hopping back the same way, and jumps out at square 1. Then the same player gets to throw the stone into number 2. This continues all the way till number 8.
- If the player fails to get the stone in the right square, the player must forfeit her turn.
- The next player then gets to have a turn.
- The player who reaches square 8 and back first wins the game.

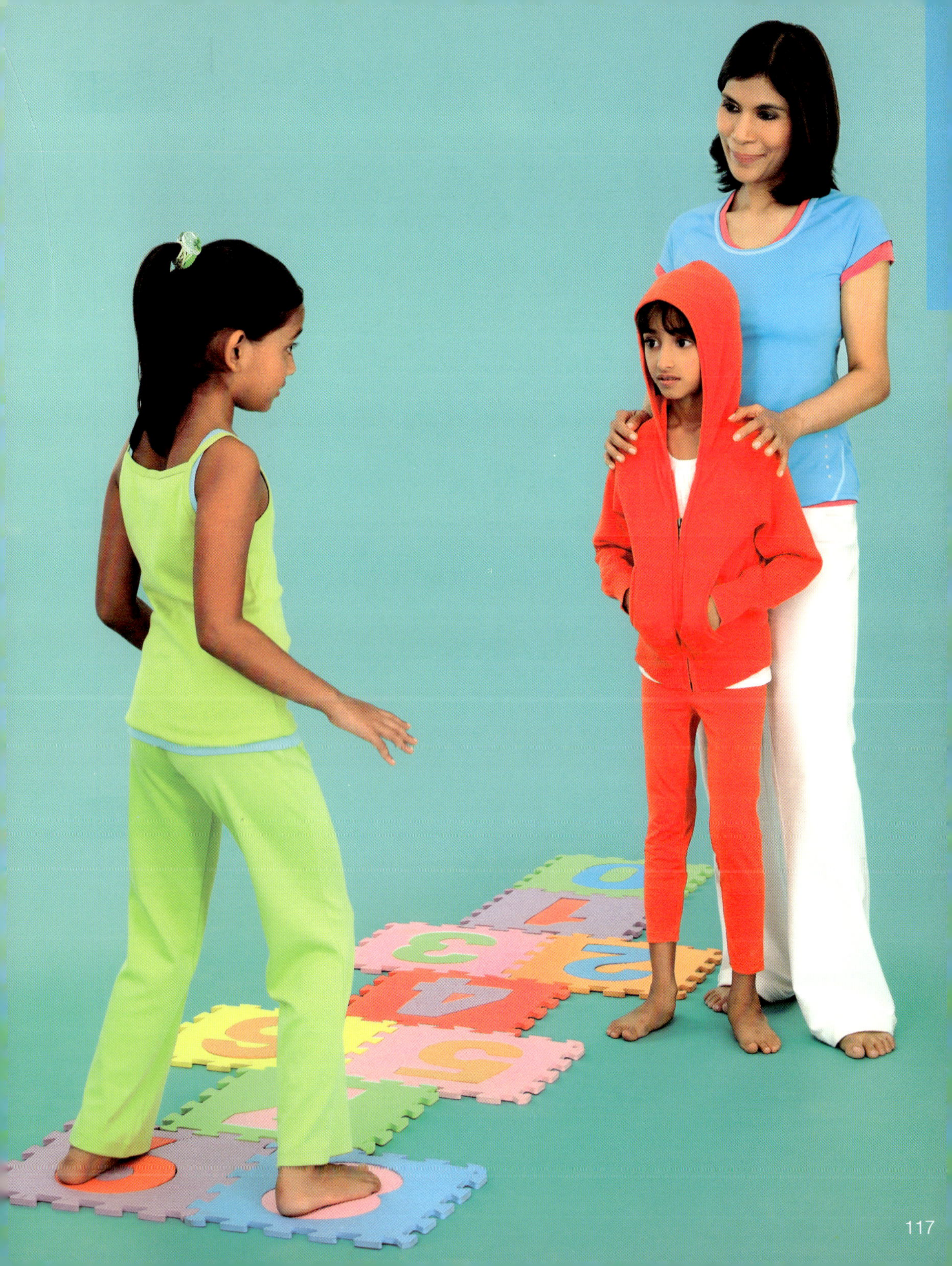

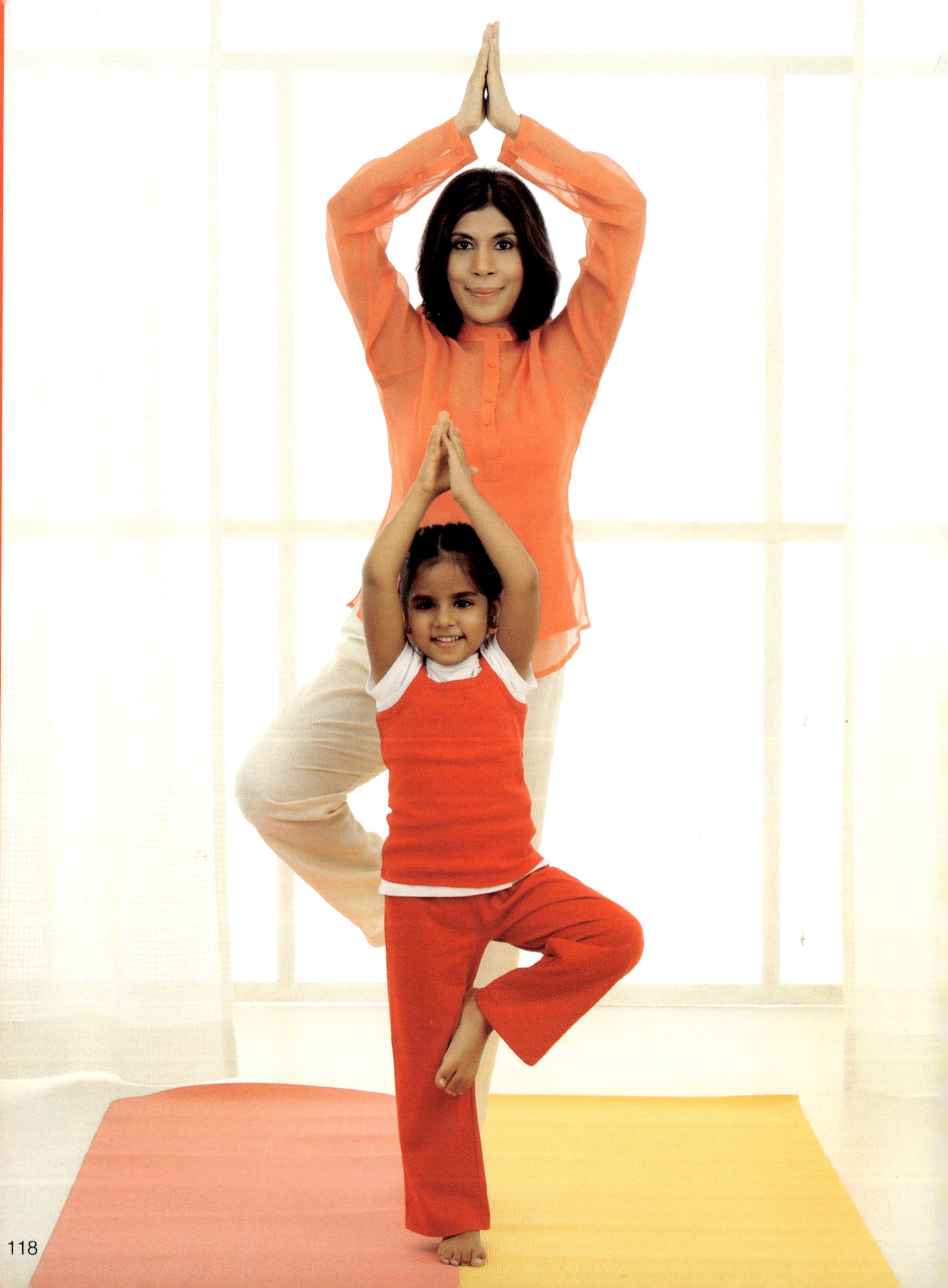

Mantra 9

Yoga is a time-tested fitness regimen that children enjoy. Simple **asanas** and "quiet time" with **breathing exercises** and meditation ensure a complete **mind and body workout** for kids of all ages.

JUNIOR YOGA

Nature has given us timeless insights into fitness and health. Working in unison with the body and mind, the science of yoga derives its postures and movements from the world around us. Relaxation and breathing techniques stem from the environment – the sun, trees, a mountain, the ocean. Children instinctively identify with animal poses, based on the movements of the locust, the lion, the cobra, the eagle, the butterfly, the monkey, and other living things. The idea is to imbibe the natural grace and beauty of life as we see it.

Children, especially very young kids, may not understand the deeper concept of yoga and meditation. However, from an early age, children can learn yoga in a practical and fun way, by doing some simple asanas and sitting down for "quiet time" as a form of meditation.

Regular yoga practice through the early years helps develop better powers of concentration and an increased attention span. An added benefit is that children will develop superior posture and balance and strengthen their bodies, both internally and externally.

Yoga also balances the body's spiritual energy centres, known as the chakras. While you do not need to go into lengthy explanations with young children, your older child may be interested in understanding more about the spiritual energy that is the root of all life forms.

yoga through the growing years

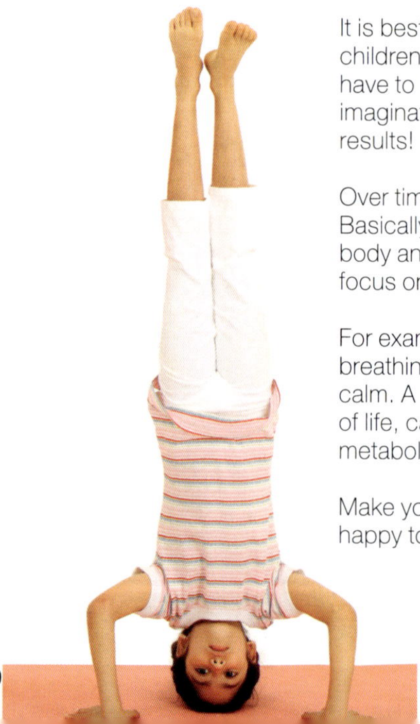

It is best to introduce your children to yoga in a phased manner. Little children are flexible, but they lack strength, so initially, the postures have to be basic. You can work with their strong sense of imagination and natural aptitude for imitation, to get the desired results!

Over time, kids can try more complex asanas and breathing control. Basically, the practice of yoga balances the energy fields within the body and creates an inner harmony. You can also help your child to focus on specific areas that need to be corrected.

For example, you could encourage your hyperactive child to perform breathing exercises or relaxation poses, to gradually become more calm. A child who tends to be sluggish, or prefers a sedentary way of life, can be encouraged to practice energetic poses to boost the metabolism and renew energy.

Make yoga a fun activity for children of all ages and they will be happy to pursue it all through their childhood.

4 to 7

4 years onwards, children can start simple asanas. This is an age when your children are going through a phase of tremendous physical and mental development. Capture their interest, by using imaginative ways to get them hooked! Think of simple stories, or try their favourite story books, as a device to introduce them to the different yoga poses.

Animal poses and movements in the form of drama keep little children entertained.

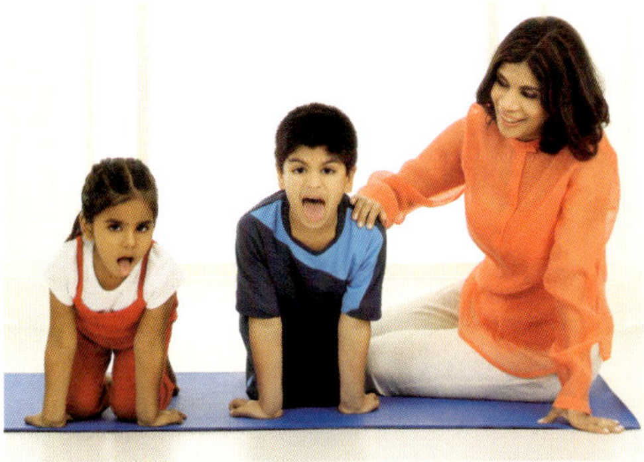

LION WITH TONGUE STICKING OUT

benefit: prevents throat congestion and strengthens throat and chest muscles

Ask your child to sit on the heels with knees apart. Hands should be placed on the floor. Then, get your child to lean forward, using the arms as support for the rest of the body. Let your kid stick the tongue out and roar like a lion.

BUTTERFLY IN A GARDEN

benefit: increases mobility of the hip joints and stretches the inner thigh

Get your child to sit with legs outstretched on the mat. Then, with knees bent, your child should bring heels of the feet in, towards the body, as close as possible. Soles of the feet should be joined together. With the spine straight, get your child to gently bounce the knees up and down in repeat movements. This resembles a butterfly flapping its wings.

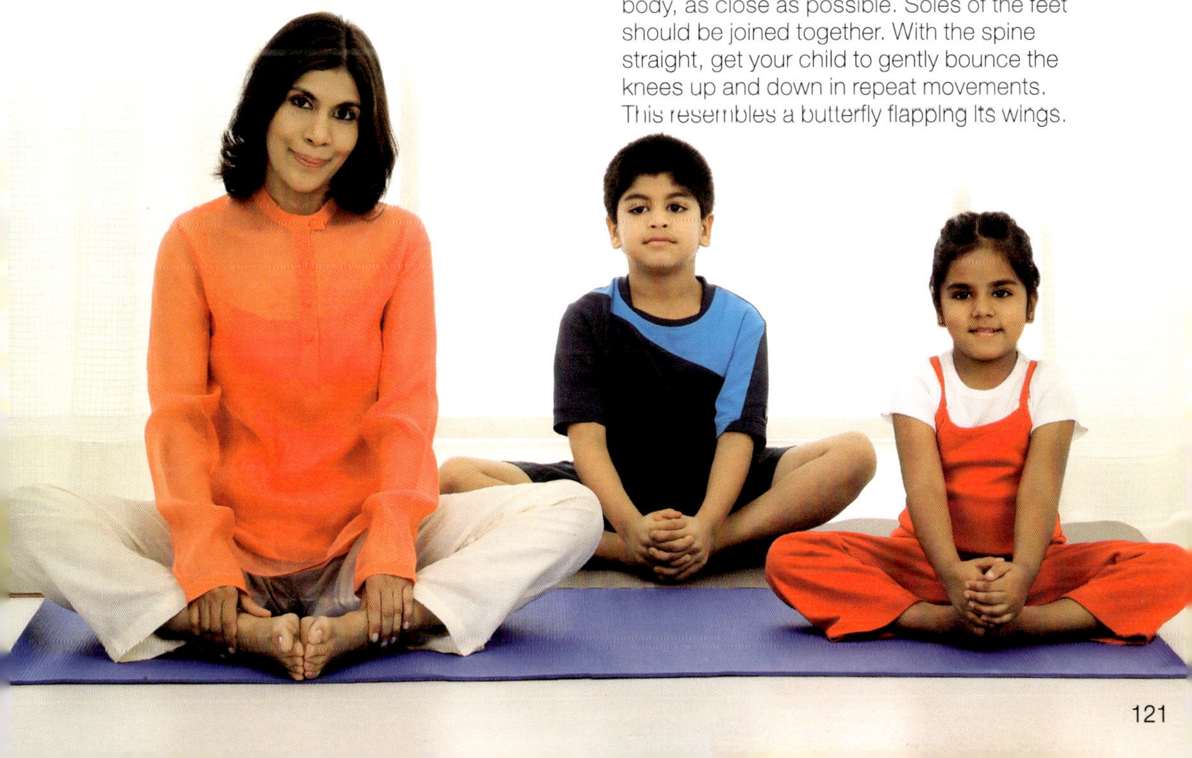

8 to 11

This is an age when yoga sessions can be more structured. Dynamic asanas, incorporating a series of different poses, can be introduced. The surya namaskar, or sun salutation, is an ideal example.

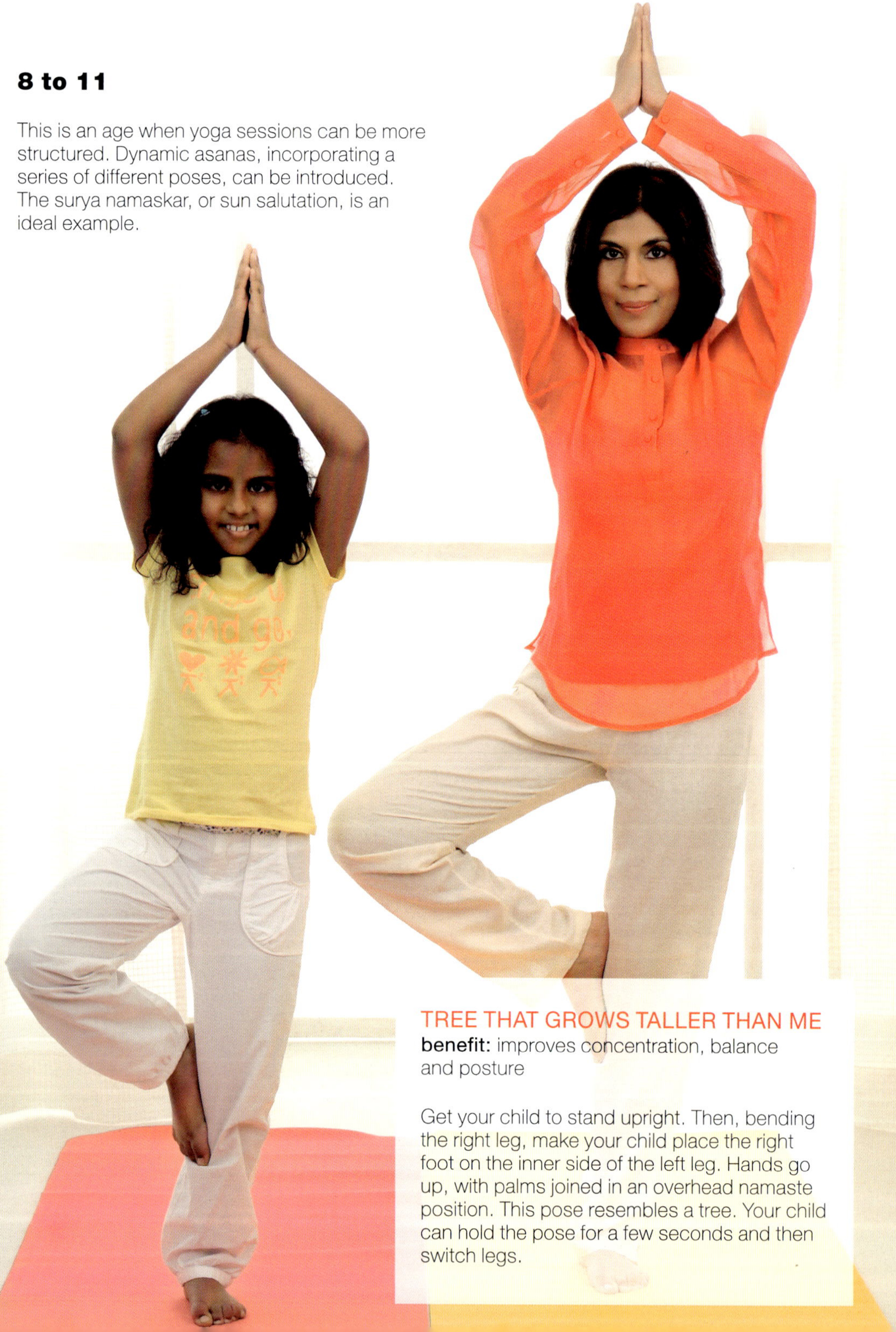

TREE THAT GROWS TALLER THAN ME

benefit: improves concentration, balance and posture

Get your child to stand upright. Then, bending the right leg, make your child place the right foot on the inner side of the left leg. Hands go up, with palms joined in an overhead namaste position. This pose resembles a tree. Your child can hold the pose for a few seconds and then switch legs.

RABBIT FINDING ITS BURROW

benefit: keeps the spine supple and stretches back of the body

Get your child to sit on the heels. With a slow movement, make your child come all the way forward, bending from the waist, until the forehead rests on the floor. Arms must be fully extended in front.

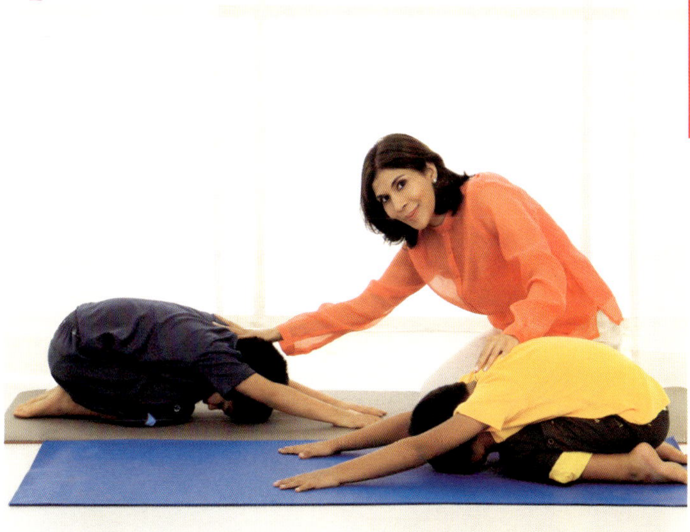

BOW LOOKING FOR THE ARROW

benefit: keeps the spine supple and stretches front of the body

Make your child lie on a mat, on the stomach. Get him or her to bend the knees and hold the ankles, or feet, with both hands. At this point, the chest must be lifted off the floor. The pose imitates a bow.

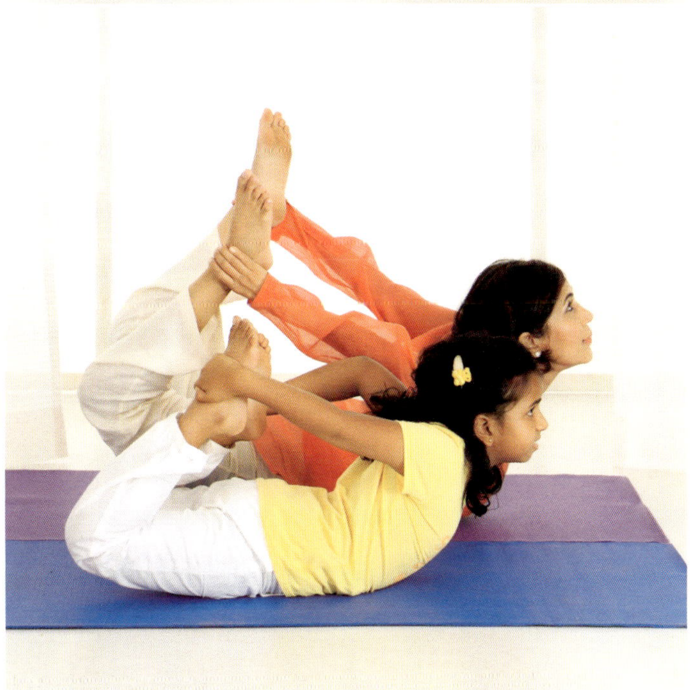

12 UPWARDS

Older children have a longer attention span, more stamina, and endurance. They are in a position to attempt slightly complex asanas, like the candle pose. This is also a good age to introduce simple breathing exercises to improve their concentration and lung capacity.

SHOULDER STAND

Get your child to lie on the back and raise both legs, bringing them up at a 90-degree angle. Then, with hands below the hips, the torso should be gradually lifted off the floor, in a smooth movement that continues till the body is resting on the shoulders. Ask your child to point the toes and keep the back as straight as possible. For first-timers, this pose will initially need your supervision.

PLOUGH POSE

From the shoulder stand position, your child can slowly lower both feet to the floor behind the head. Legs should be straight and toes should touch the floor.

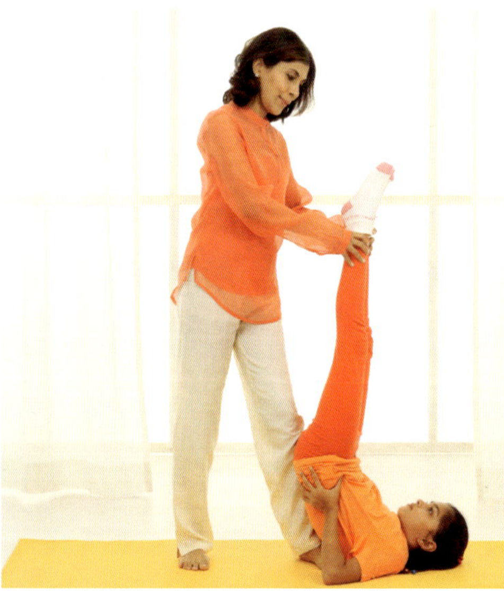

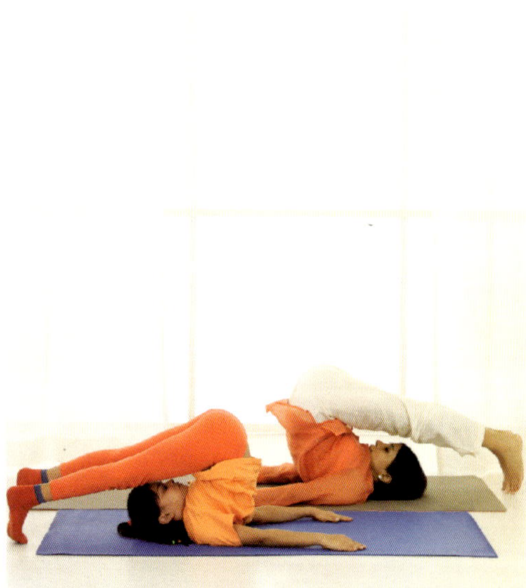

BALANCING STICK POSE

Get your teenager to stand tall, raise the arms up over the head, and lean forward. The body should then be propelled in a forward bend, and simultaneously, one leg should be lifted off the floor. The level of the hands and the leg should form a straight line, parallel to the floor. Repeat with the other leg.

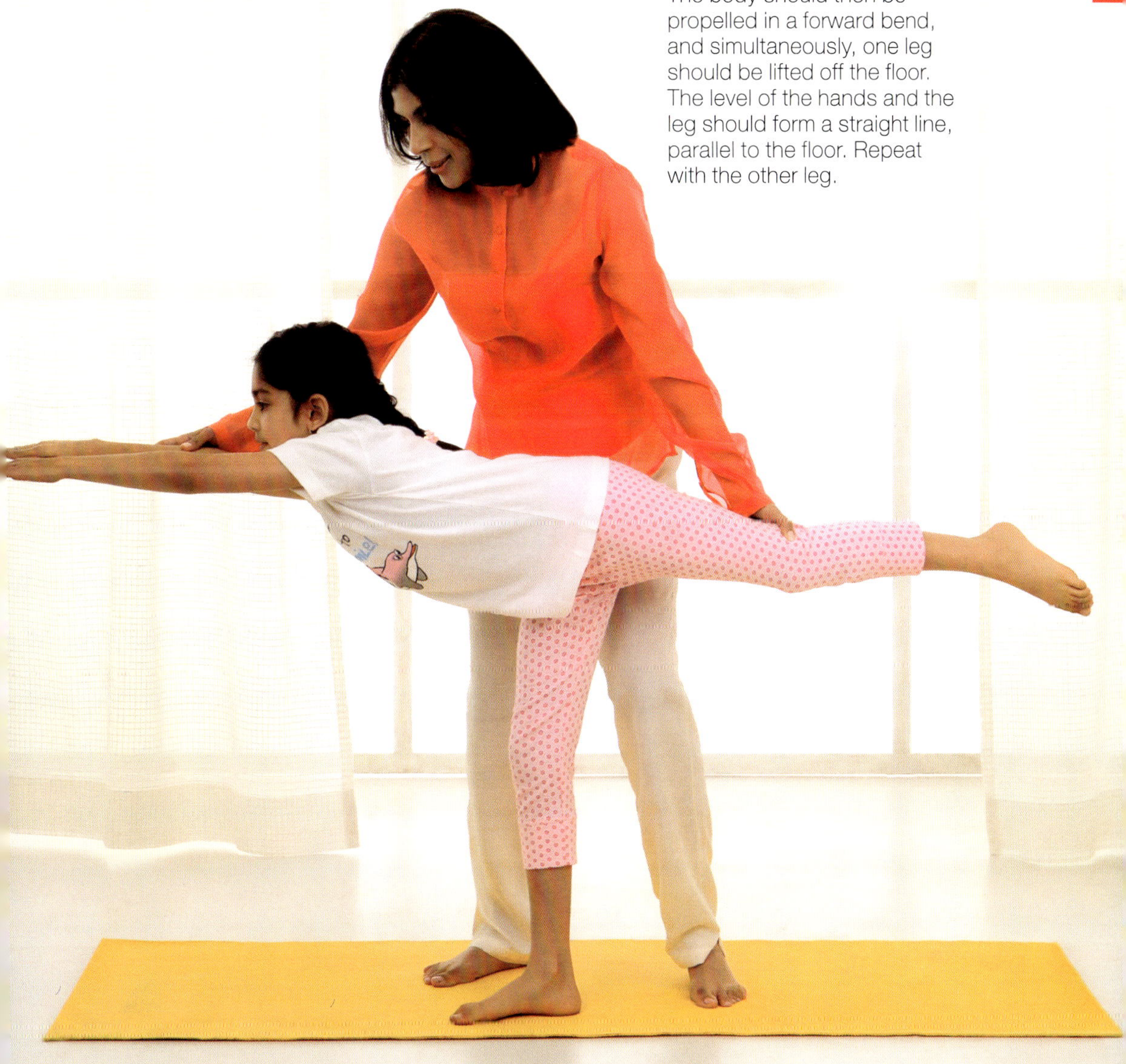

the yoga routine

Yoga poses invigorate body and mind, stretch the spine and stimulate the internal organs. The body's natural energy channels are activated, to ensure energy blockages are removed and the chakras remain in balance.

How often to practice?

Daily practice is ideal, but even if your child can manage three yoga sessions in a week, it is extremely beneficial for the body, mind and spirit.

Where to practice?

Yoga can be practiced anywhere, indoors or outdoors, as long as it is a quiet, peaceful environment. If your child is indoors, make sure that there is adequate ventilation within the room.

Yoga gear

It's important to make sure your child wears loose, comfortable clothing. In addition, he or she will need a yoga mat, rug, blanket or a carpet, to practice many of the prone positions.

Holding a yoga pose

Ask your child to hold each posture between 10 to 60 seconds.

I have included here some common poses that your children will enjoy practicing. The sequence can be completed in the order that it is presented. Help your children to follow the simple instructions I have provided for each pose.

You can either participate with your children, or instruct them to practice independently – but make sure they learn to do the poses in a correct manner.

The instructions are easy to follow, enabling you to spend quality time with your children.

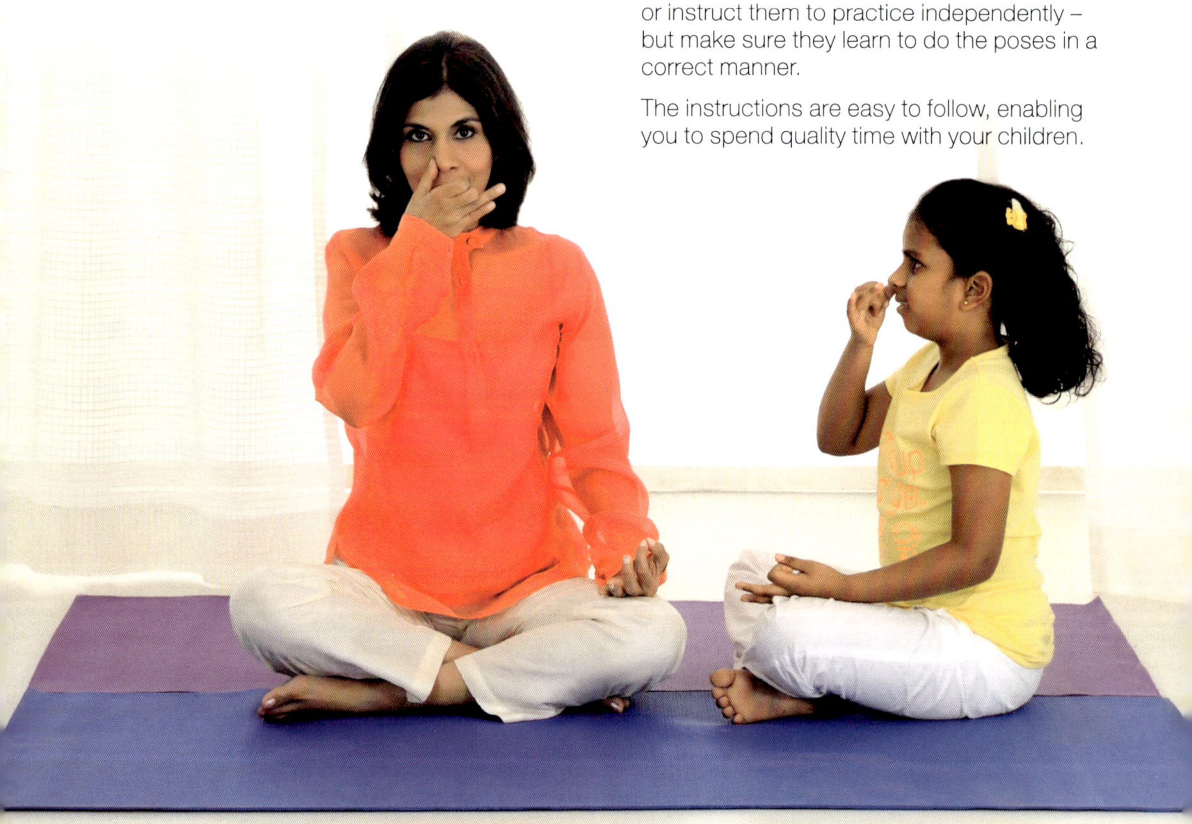

palm tree

benefit: stretches and strengthens the torso

See how well your child can imitate a palm tree, by standing tall and strong, and pretending to 'sway' in the wind.

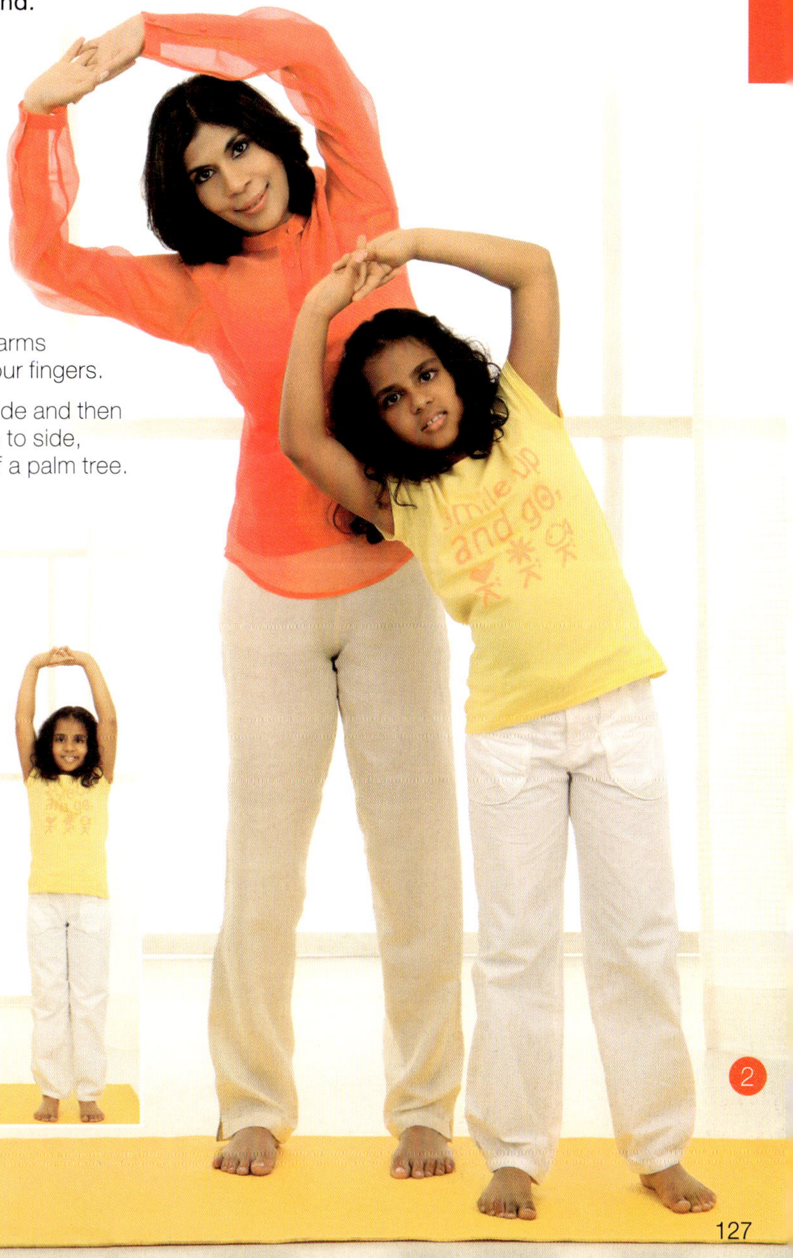

1. Stand upright, raise your arms overhead and interlock your fingers.
2. Now stretch to the right side and then to the left, sway from side to side, imitating the movement of a palm tree.

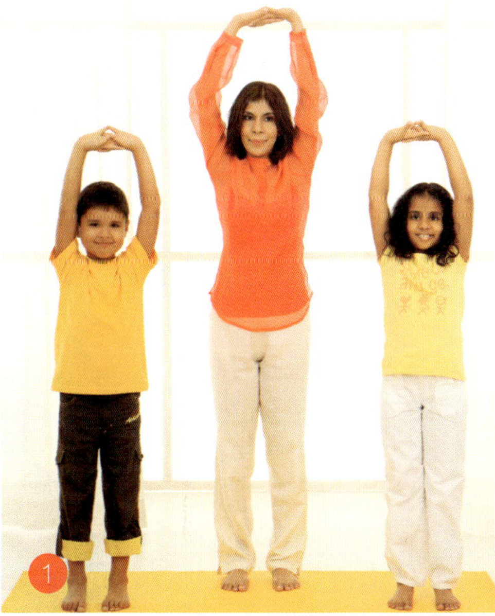

1

2

triangle pose

benefit: regulates the digestive system and massages internal organs, such as the liver

Can your child position the body in such a way that it forms 3 triangles?

1. Stand with your feet wide apart and hands stretched outwards at shoulder level, parallel to the floor.
2. Stretch the left hand up and bend down to the right side. Look up towards the left hand. Return to starting position and switch sides.

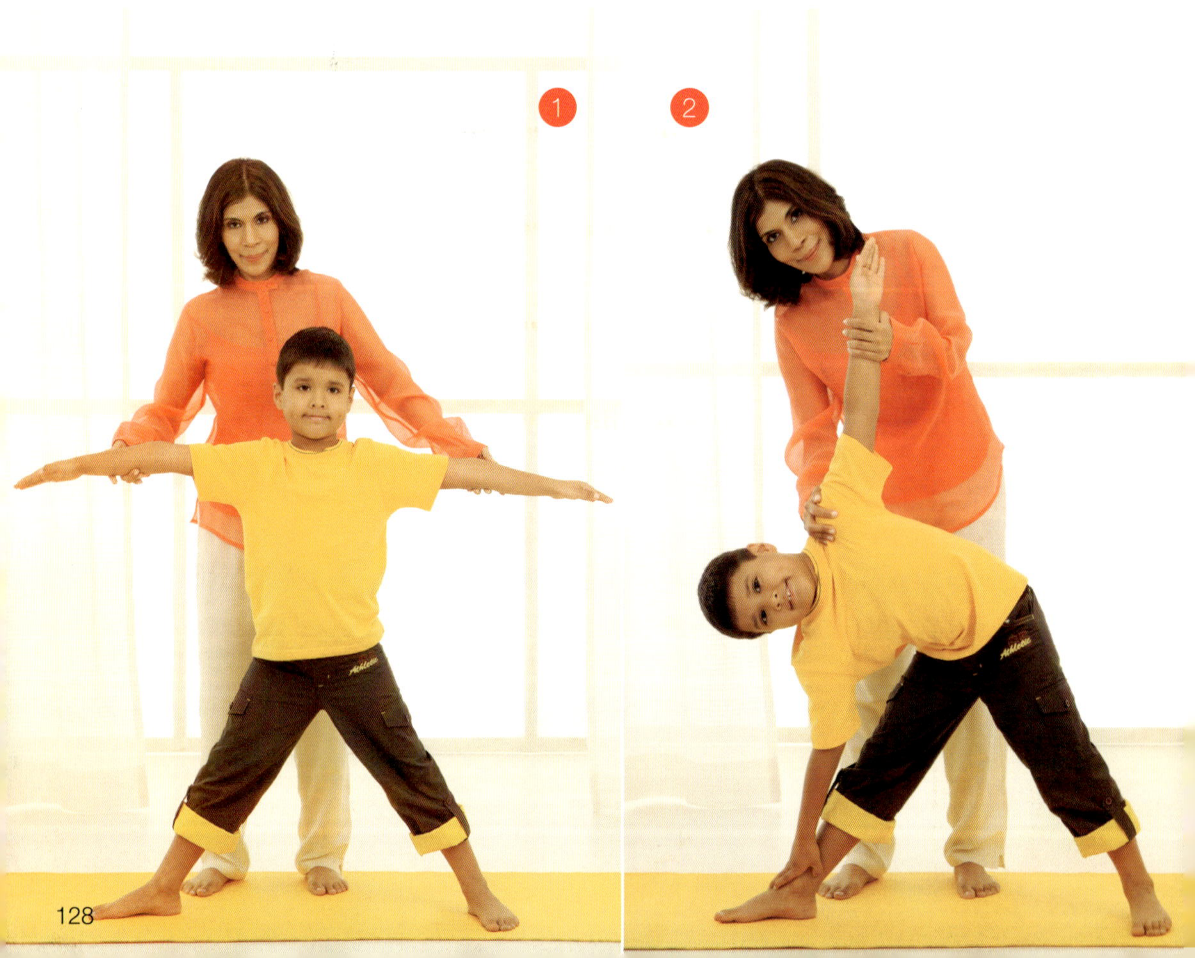

the dancer

benefit: strengthens the leg muscles and improves stability and concentration

This pose resembles a graceful dancer.

1. Stand tall.
2. Stretch your left hand up, bend your right knee back and hold the ankle with your right hand. Slowly tilt your body forward and raise your leg backward. Return to starting position and switch legs.

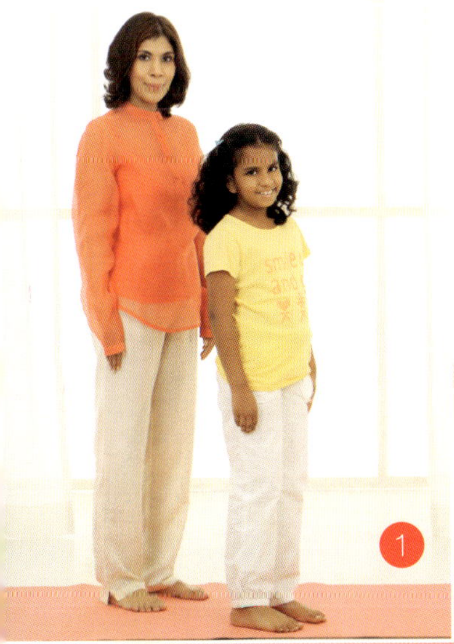

1

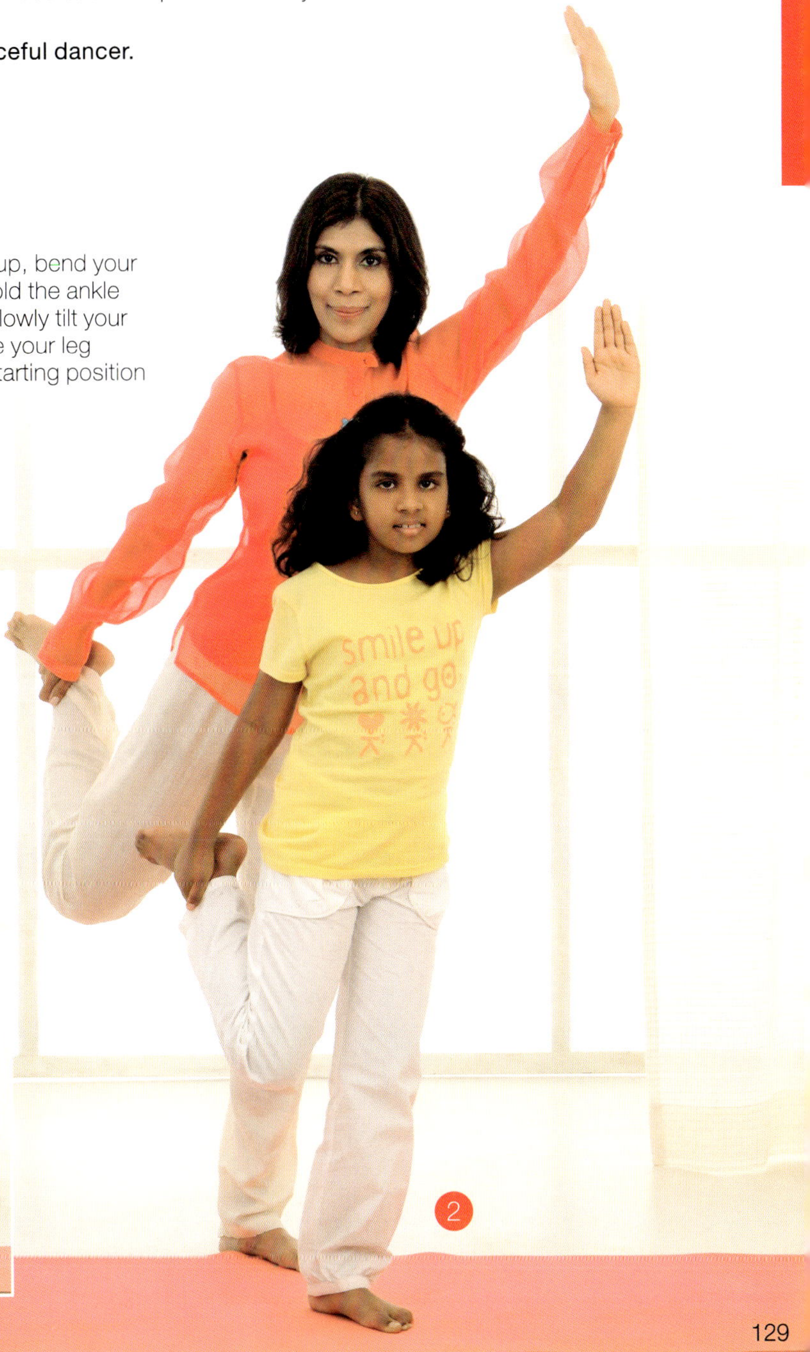

2

the boat

benefit: strengthens the abdominals and improves stability

Can your child hold this pose? It's a delicate balancing act that requires abdominal strength to do properly!

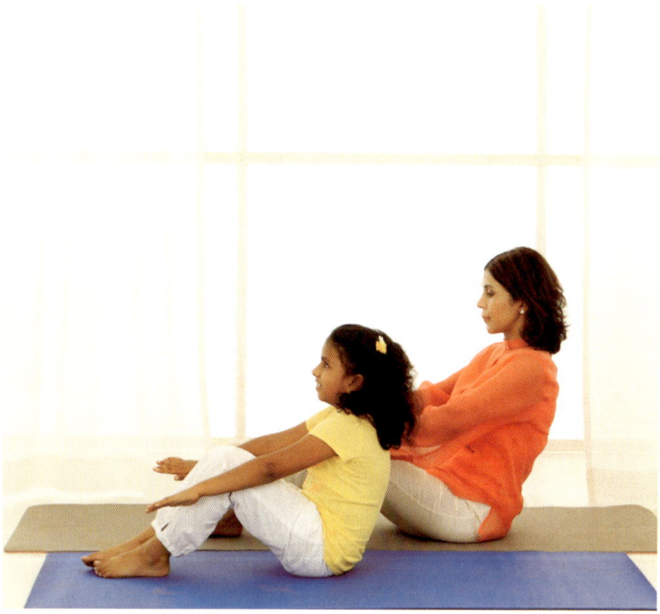

1. Sit with your knees bent.

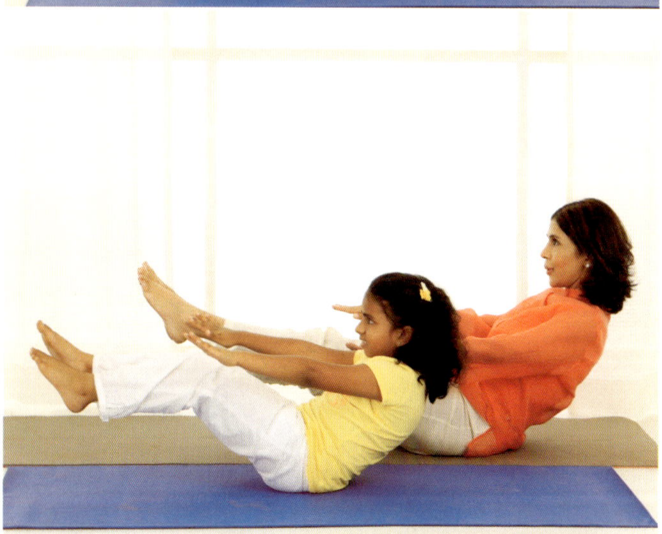

2. Lean back and lift your legs off the floor until you are in a boat position. Hold this position, balancing on your tail bone.

the bridge

benefit: strengthens the back, stretches the torso and improves stability

This position strengthens and stretches the torso simultaneously.

1. Lie on your back with your knees bent.
2. Lift your hips and back off the floor like a bridge position.

2

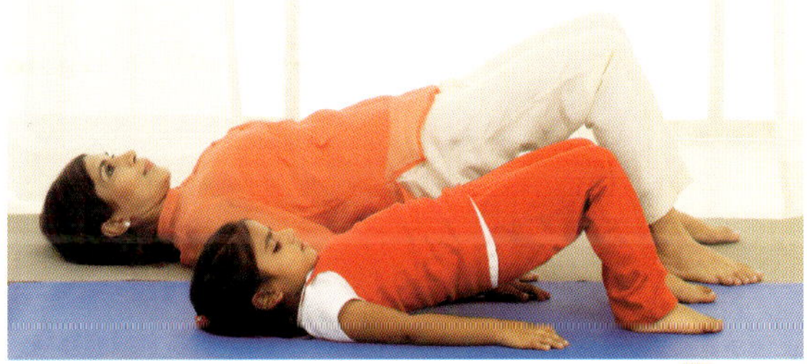

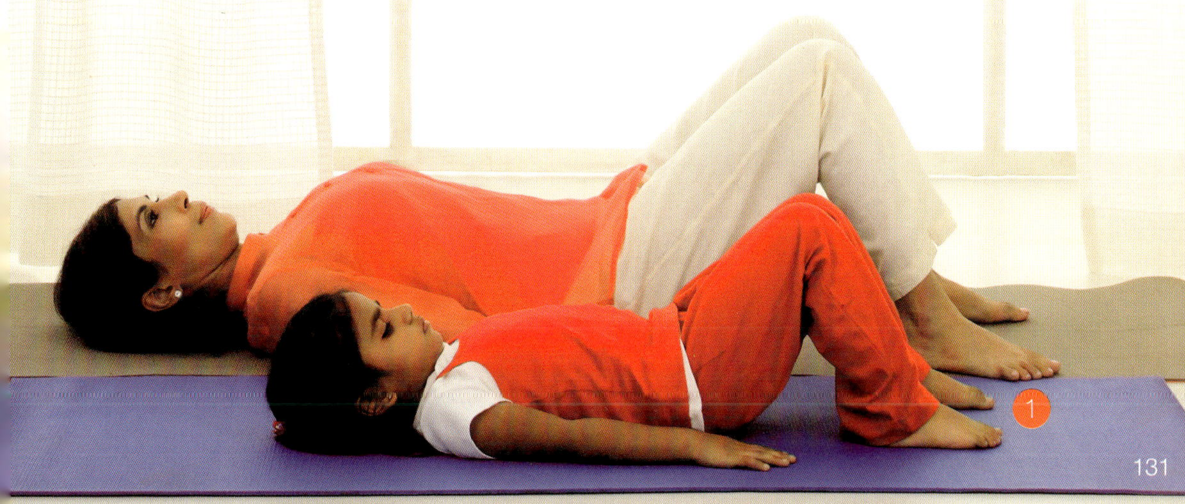

1

knee hug

benefit: stretches the hip and lower back

This comforting position resembles a knee hug and relaxes the hips and back.

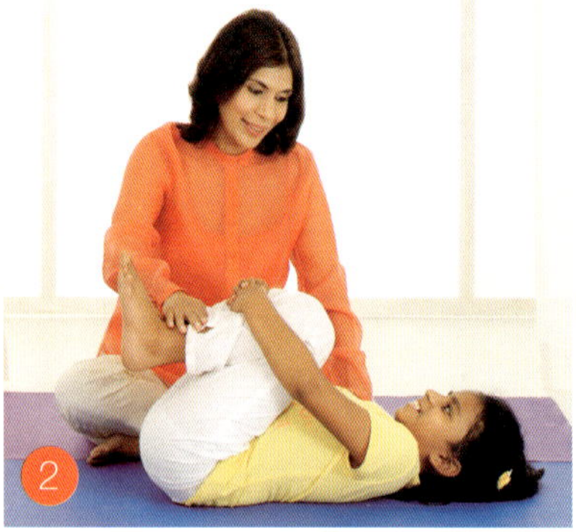

2

1. Lie on your back with knees bent.
2. Lift legs off the floor, draw knees towards chest.

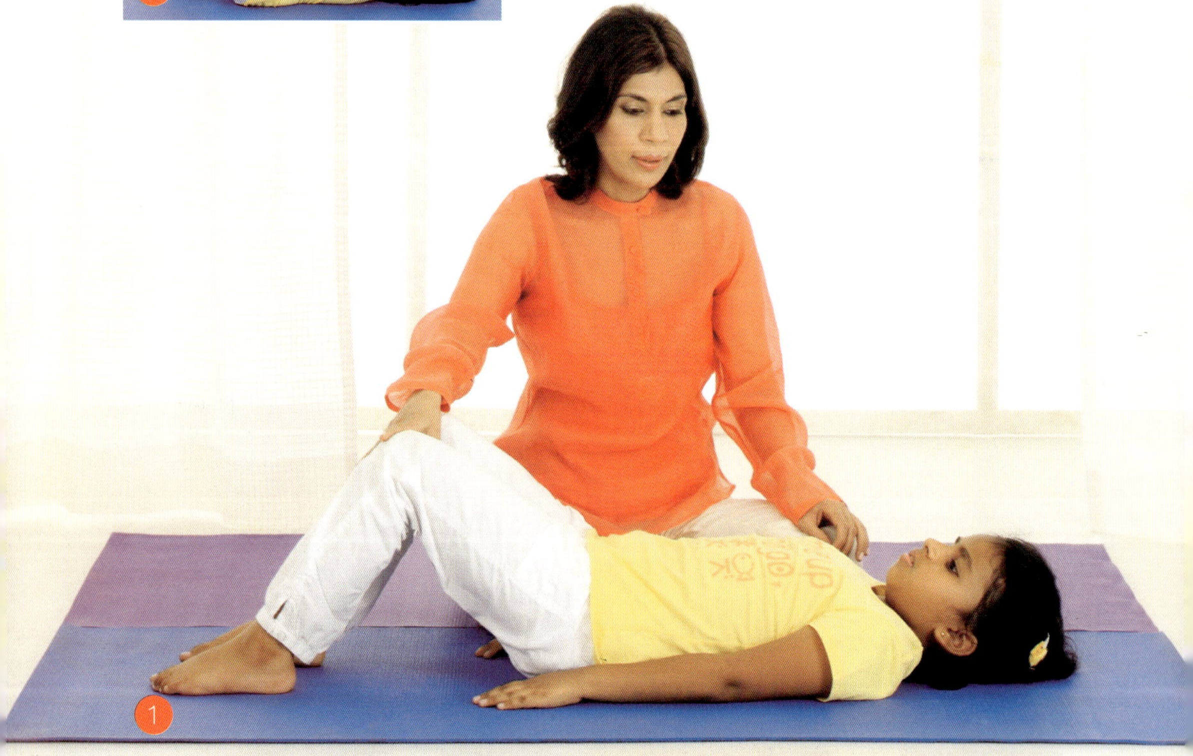

1

seated twist

benefit: stretches the spine, improves digestion and relieves constipation

The right-to-left and left-to-right twisting movement greatly improves mobility of the spine.

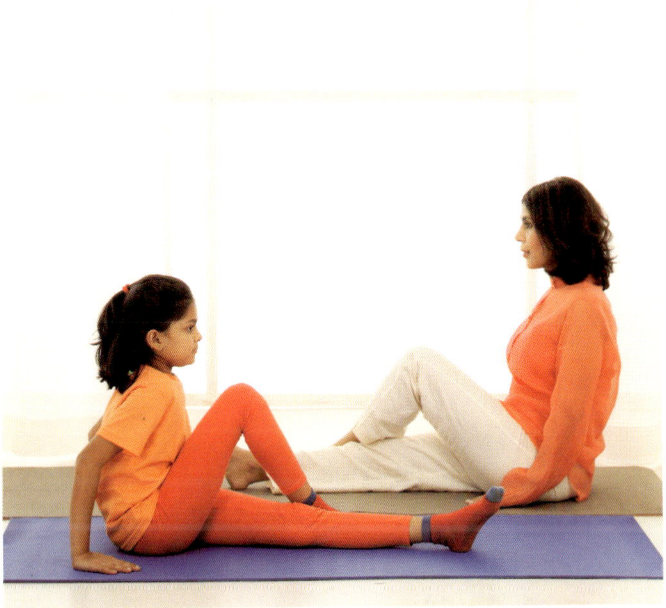

1. Sit with your legs extended out in front of you. Bend the right knee and take the foot over the left knee.

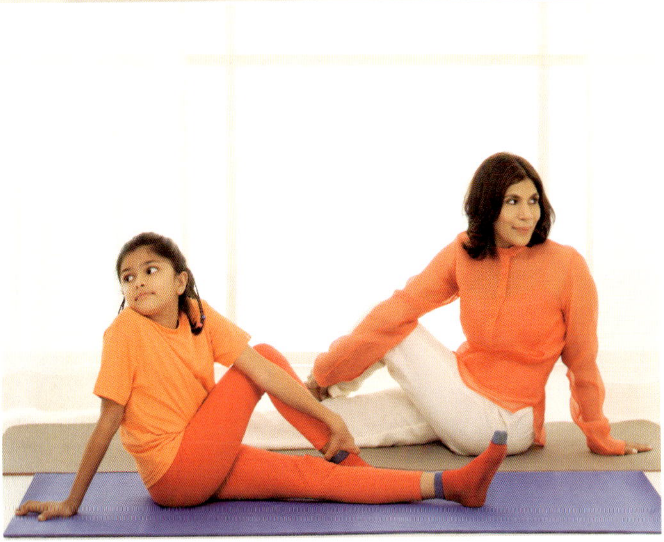

2. Bring the left arm and elbow over the right knee. Now twist your torso to the right, turning your head as far back as possible. Return to starting position and switch sides.

the cobra

benefit: massages abdominal muscles and strengthens the spine

This pose resembles a cobra when it lifts its hood up and hisses, as if it's about to strike!

1. Lie with your abs resting on the mat. Place your palms flat on the mat, facing downwards, just below your shoulders.
2. Now slowly lift your head and chest and arch your back. Try not to place too much weight on your hands, but use your back muscles to lift your chest up.

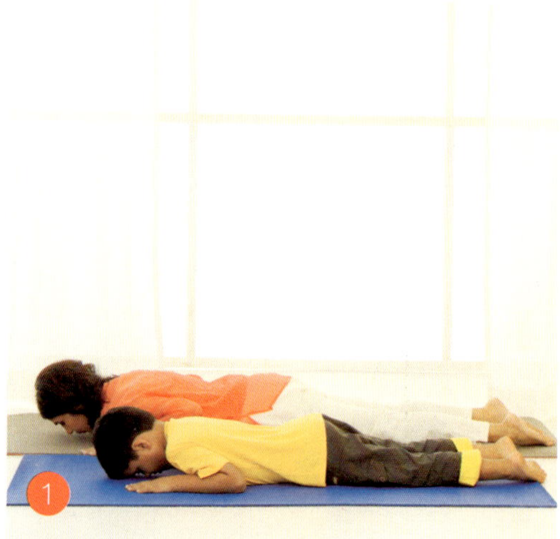

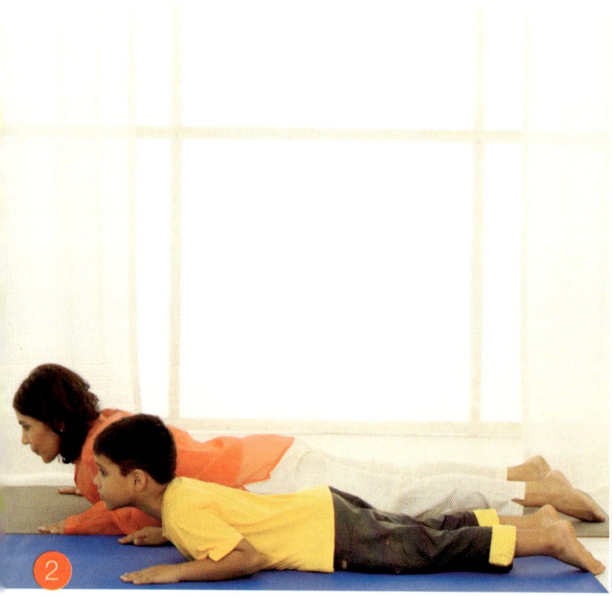

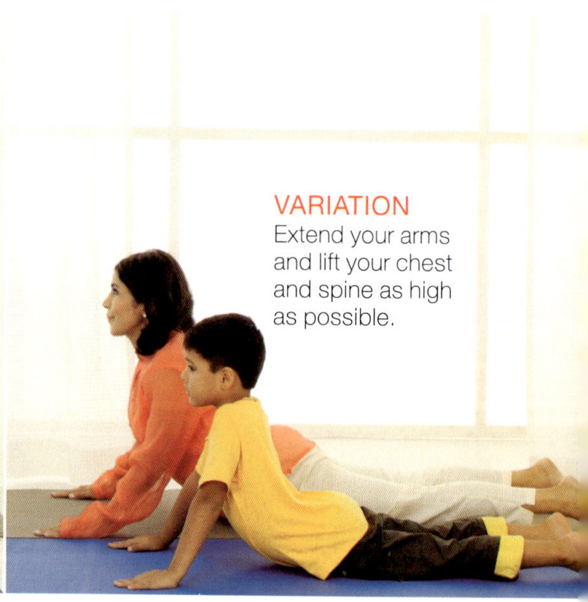

VARIATION
Extend your arms and lift your chest and spine as high as possible.

the cat-camel

benefit: releases spinal stress

Imitate a cat and then a camel. Can your child dip the spine like a cat and then lift it up like the hump of a camel?

1. Kneel down with hands placed on the mat, like a cat on all fours. Place your hands directly below your shoulders. Now lift your tailbone up towards the ceiling and lift your head up to the ceiling, so that your back becomes a shallow "U" shape.
2. Now, raise the centre of your back up, like the hump of a camel and roll your head towards your chest. Make the movements as fluid as possible.

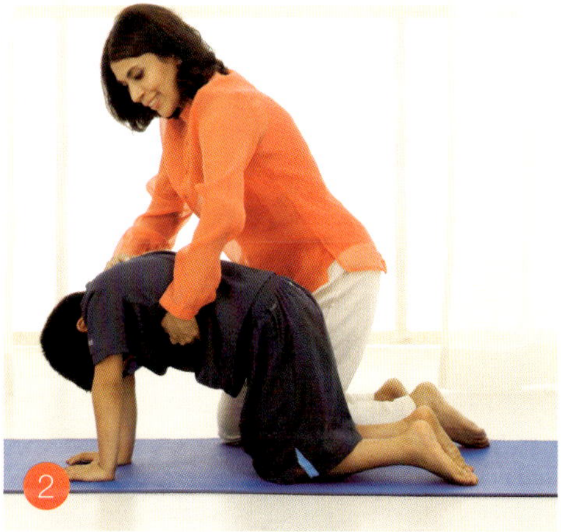

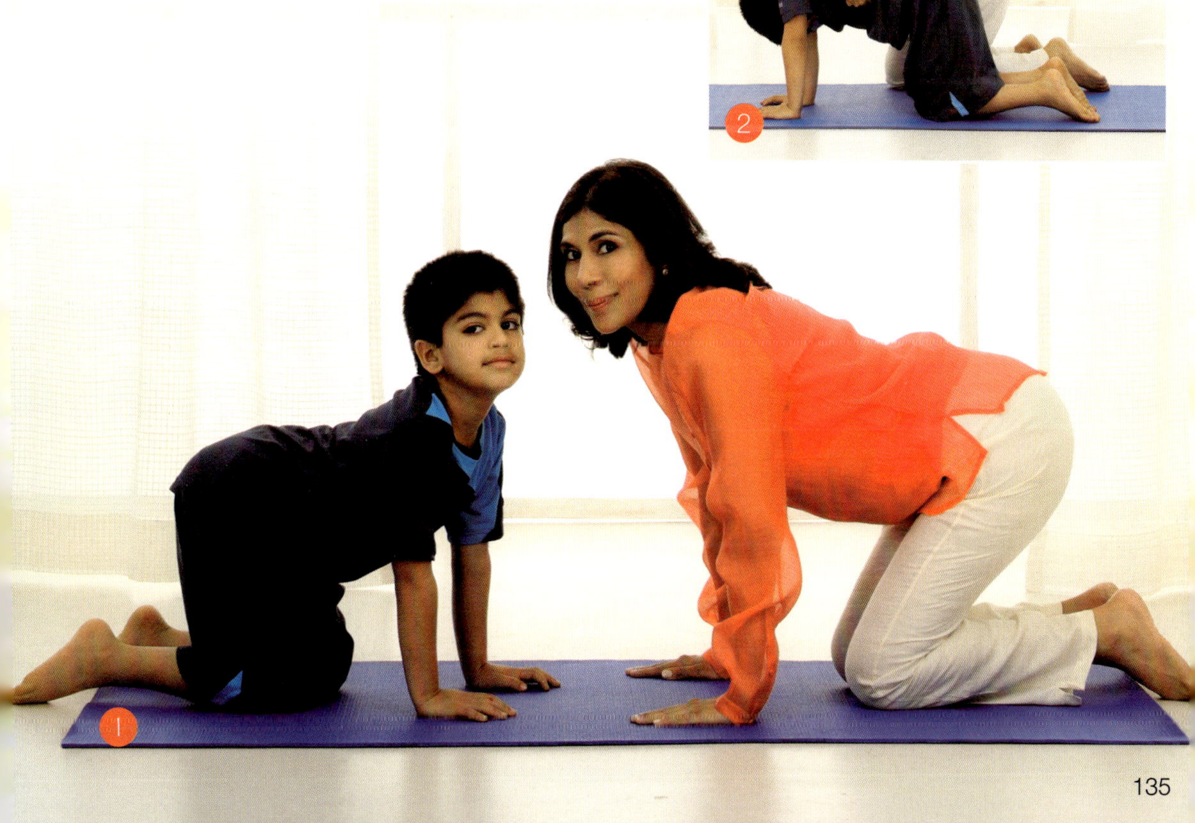

the lying down spinal twist

benefit: improves flexibility of the spine and strengthens abdominal organs

A really relaxing twist!

1. Lie on your back, bend knees and bring them close together.
2. Drop both your bent legs to the right, and look in the opposite direction, hold. Then, keeping both knees together, centre your legs and drop legs to the left side, looking in the opposite direction.

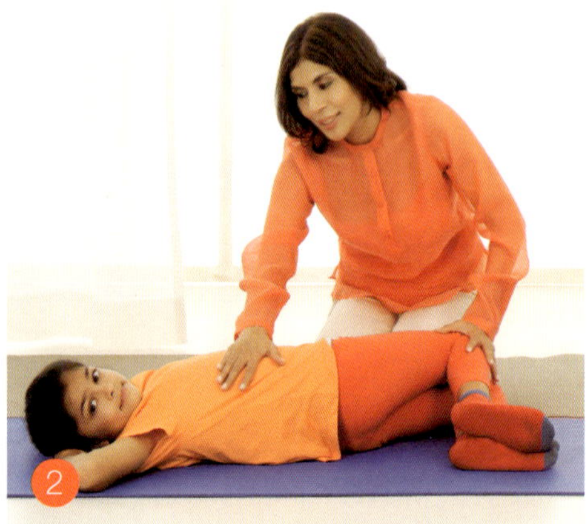

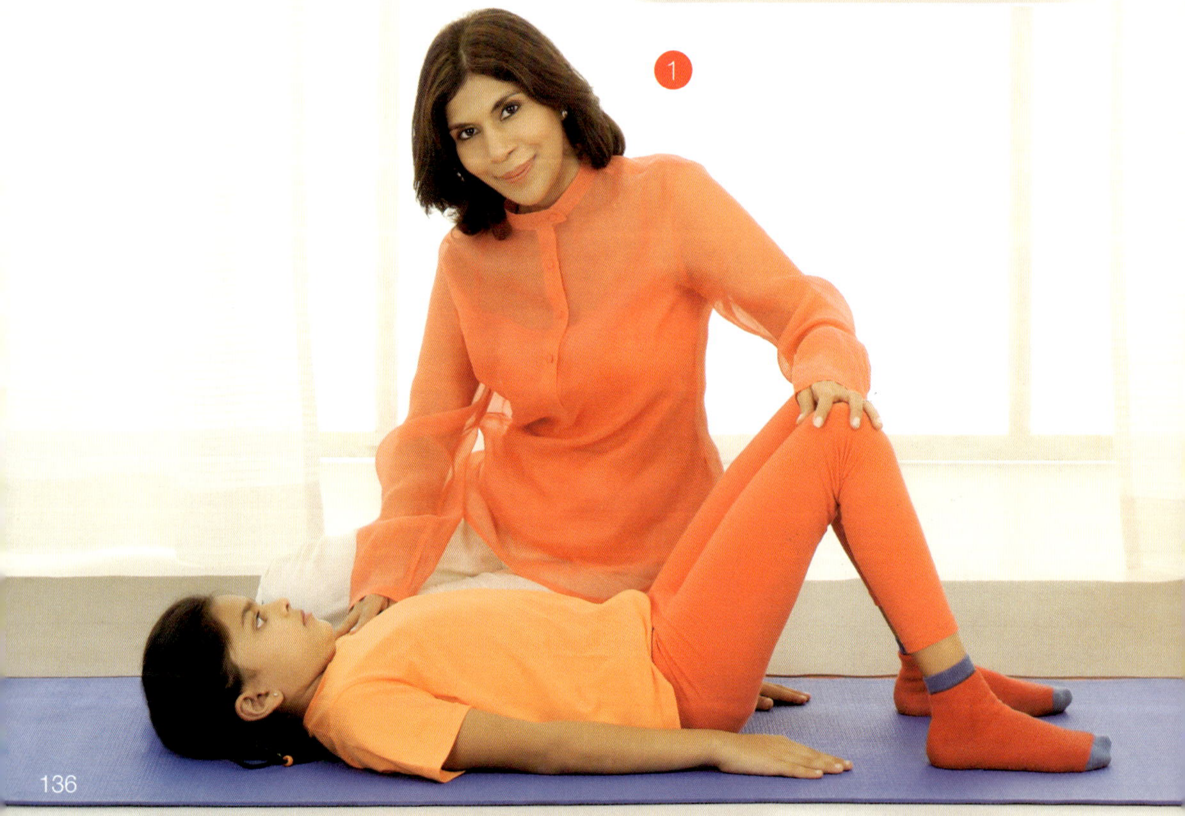

breathing & relaxation

belly breathing : how to breathe using the diaphragm to is fullest

1. Lie on your back. Place a small toy on your tummy. Inhale, and fill your belly with air, so the toy rises.
2. Then exhale, so that your toy sinks down again.

YOGIC SLEEP

This is the last pose, a great way to finish off the yoga routine and get your child to feel relaxed and rejuvenated.

1. Lie on the mat, with arms and legs loose, slightly away from the body.

2. The eyes are closed and the mind is relaxed.

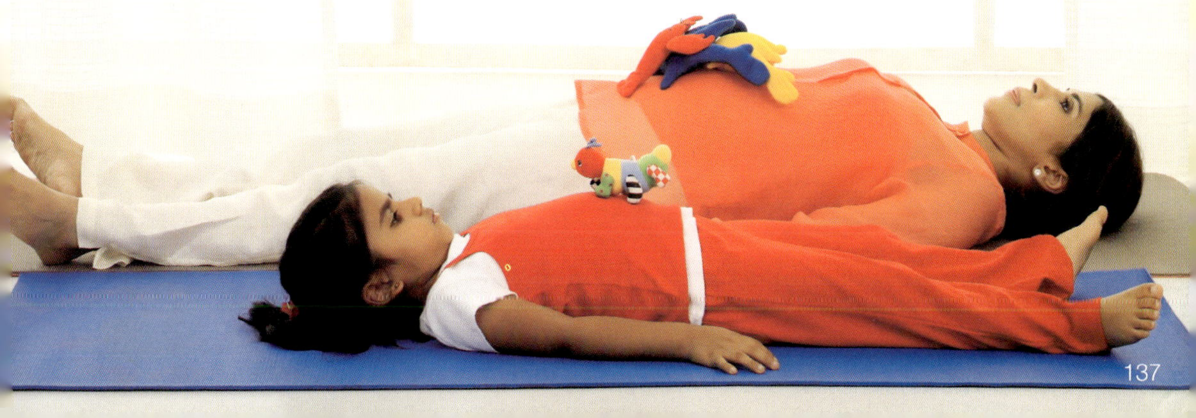

the 7 chakras

Mantra 9 covers the seven chakras, as this is an integral part of the science of yoga.

Chakra means 'wheel' in Sanskrit. There are seven chakras - the wheels of energy - in the astral body. Six of them are found along the spine and the seventh is located at the crown of the head.

Chakras are powerful energy centres in the body. Although they are invisible to the eye, these wheels of spiritual energy balance the body and spirit. The chakras store dynamic energy known to yogis in India as kundalini, to the Chinese as Ch'i, and to the Japanese as Ki.

Each chakra spins in a clockwise direction and is depicted by a colour. These whirling vortices of energy glow with the light of the spectrum, from red at the base, to violet at the crown. Each of the seven chakras has a unique characteristic and has a vital role in our physical body as well as in our consciousness.

The three lower chakras correlate to basic primary needs, those of survival, procreation and will. The four higher chakras correlate to the psychological make up and represent higher spiritual qualities such as love, compassion and understanding.

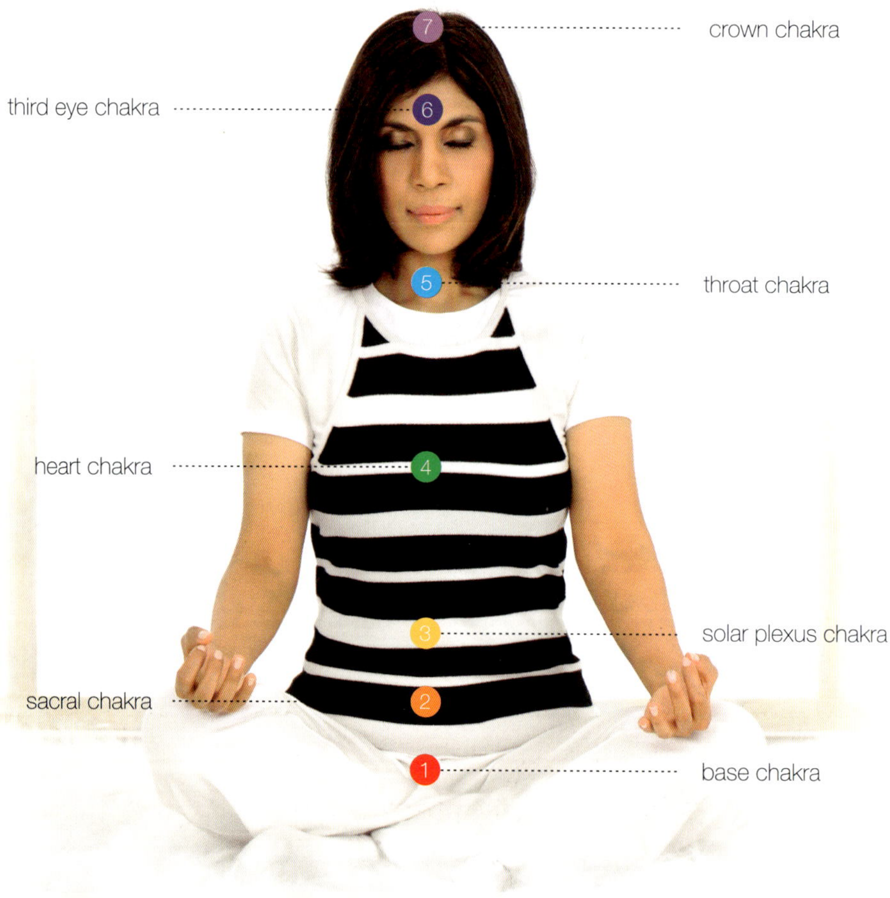

SEVEN CHAKRAS

CHAKRA	COLOUR	BODY SYSTEM
1. Muladhara		
base chakra	red	elimination, lymph system
Affirmation: "I am connected to mother earth and feel secure and protected."		
2. Svadhishtana		
sacral chakra	orange	digestive, reproductive systems
Affirmation: "I am worthy of love. Life offers me everything I need for that journey".		
3. Manipura		
solar plexux chakra	yellow	intestines, liver
Affirmation: "I know I am becoming the best person I can be."		
4. Anahata		
heart chakra	green	heart and lungs
Affirmation: "I love myself for who I am and the potential within me."		
5. Vishuddha		
throat chakra	blue	throat
Affirmation: "My voice, thoughts and speech are filled with conviction."		
6. Ajna		
third eye chakra	indigo	forehead
Affirmation: "The answers to all my questions lie within me."		
7. Sahasrara		
crown chakra	violet	brain
Affirmation: "I release all limited thoughts and lift myself up to levels of awareness".		

Let's end with a divine hymn, the Gayatri Mantra. Children will love the chanting and the universal message it holds.

THE GAYATRI MANTRA

OM BHUR BHUVAH SVAHA	Help us to know your infinite glory
TAT SAVITUR VARENYAM	Oh Lord, creator and energizer of the whole universe
BHARGO DESVASYA DHIMAHI	The giver of happiness Who is pure and the purifier
DHIYO YO NAHA PHRACHODAYAT	Let us embrace the wisdom Of the Divinity.
OM SHANTI SHANTI SHANTI	Om peace, peace peace

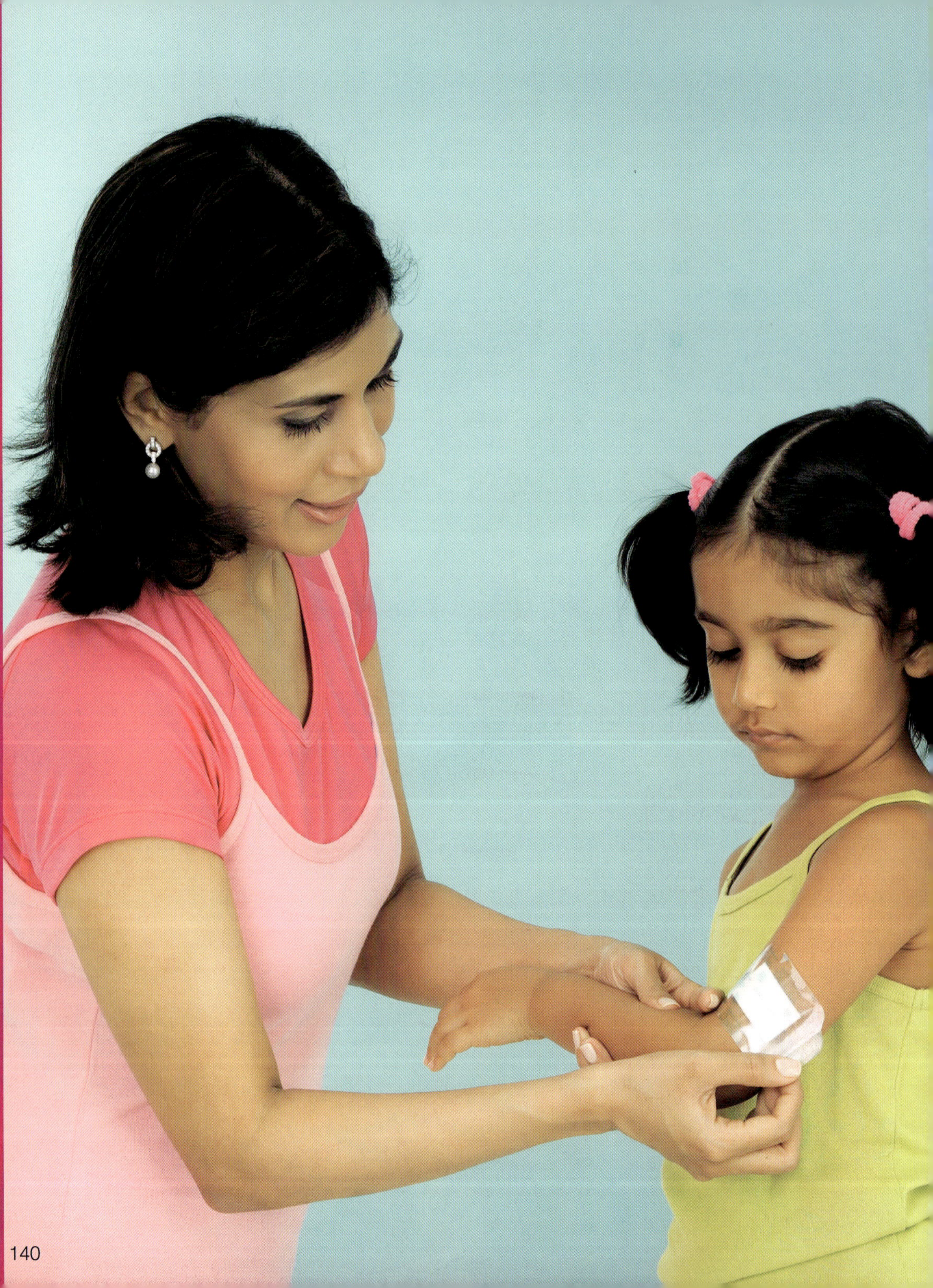

Mantra 10

For minor maladies and mishaps, **First Aid** comes to the rescue. The use of First Aid techniques and **home remedies** for common children's ailments are detailed in this chapter.

FIRST-AID: TO THE RESCUE

When you are looking after children, you have to expect the unexpected! They need your help for small maladies and mishaps, which often require prompt attention. This chapter has easy-to-follow guidelines on common problems, all very much a part of growing up. I have identified 10 of the most frequently-cited problems and offered an immediate course of action for each of these. Do keep in mind, it is always best to consult your physician for further guidance and medical advice.

In most cases, all you need to do is keep a cool head and follow the guidelines, to help your child recover smoothly.

FIRST AID KIT FOR HOME USE

Families with young children should always be equipped with a First Aid Kit at home. It is an essential resource, to be kept in readiness for emergency situations. A fully-equipped First Aid Kit can minimize the impact of accidents and injuries and save precious minutes in times of crisis.

Look for a good quality ready-made kit from the chemist, or make up your own. Label it FIRST AID in bold letters and store it in a safe, dry place. The list below covers basic must haves in your First-Aid Kit.

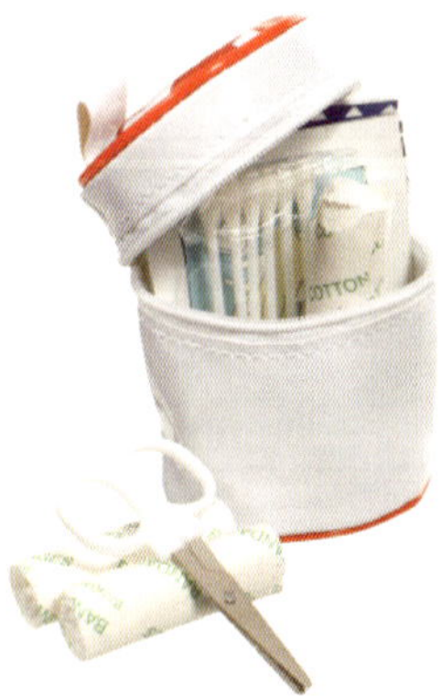

- pair of scissors
- pair of tweezers
- bottle of antiseptic solution (like Dettol or Savlon)
- antiseptic cream
- band-aids
- bandages (1 - 2 inches wide)
- cotton wool
- adhesive tape
- sterile gauze pads
- digital thermometer
- petroleum jelly
- common medications prescribed by physician
- phone numbers of your physician, hospital, and a close friend or relative

MAINTAINING A FIRST AID KIT

- If you use an item, be sure to replace it as soon as possible.
- Check contents at least once a year and replace expired items.
- Store kit high in a cupboard, out of the reach of small children.
- Make sure the kit remains clean and dry.
- Ensure kit is clearly labeled, with all items within also labeled, allowing easy access to items even if you are not present.

1 allergies | 2 bites, scratches & stings | 3 bleeding | 4 blisters
5 diarrhoea | 6 fainting | 7 nose bleeds | 8 sprains
9 bumps & bruises | 10 home remedies

1 allergies

An allergic reaction occurs when the body's immune system treats a normally harmless substance as if it were a foreign invader. Symptoms of allergies can vary from child to child.

Children may develop allergies at any time. Common triggers include drugs and medicines, foods, pollen, insect bites and stings. Sometimes, an allergic reaction could manifest itself as an asthma attack. Common foods that may cause allergic reactions in children are milk, eggs, nuts, soya products, fish, shellfish and wheat.

TYPICAL ALLERGY SYMPTOMS

- a red, blotchy spreading skin rash
- nausea or vomiting
- swelling of a body part
- puffy or watery eyes
- sneezing and runny nose
- abdominal pain
- diarrhoea
- intense itching at the site of contact, or around the mouth

For mild symptoms, anti-histamine drugs may help. If your child is suffering an asthma attack, use an inhaler for relief.

Always seek prompt medical attention.

2 bites, scratches & stings

Any type of animal bite or scratch requires instant attention. It is important to reduce the chances of infection. Usually, insect bites cause mild discomfort for a little while. A snake bite, however, is serious and you need to call an ambulance.

Human bites should immediately be treated with antibiotics

IMMEDIATE ACTION: You can use an ice pack to reduce pain and swelling

Always seek prompt medical attention.

Animal bite **ALERT!**

- Puncture marks from teeth
- Scratches
- Pain, redness & swelling around the wound

3 bleeding

Bleeding could occur with any wound, big or small. A break in the skin causes the blood to flow out, sometimes gushing out in an alarming way.

You need to keep calm and respond to the situation.

WHAT YOU CAN DO

1. Use a dressing pad or use your hand, to press firmly over the wound.
2. Keep injured limb above the level of the heart to reduce blood flow to the injured part. This helps to staunch the flow of blood and minimize blood loss.
3. When blood flow lessens, secure a dressing over the area with a moderately tight bandage.

> Bleeding **ALERT!**
> - A wound with external bleeding
> - Bruising and other signs of injury

Always seek prompt medical attention.

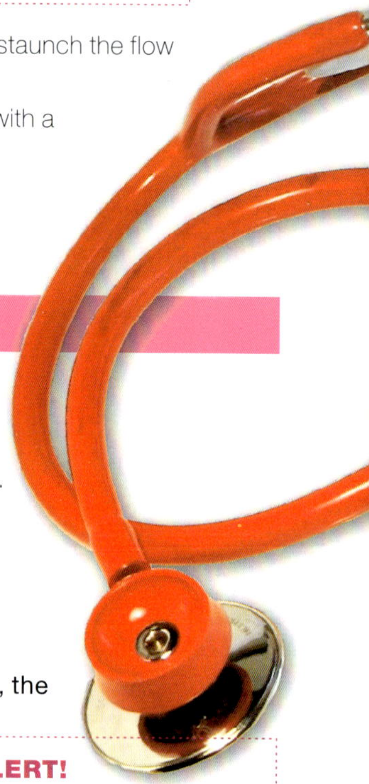

4 blisters

A blister is a swelling on the skin, with fluid inside. It is usually painful to touch. Blisters can result from infections, chemicals or allergies. Typical blisters are due to new shoes, sunburn, or touching something very hot. Most blisters heal by themselves.

If the blister area bursts spontaneously, cover it with a sterile dressing. In case of friction in the blistered area, like shoe bite, for example, you may need to protect it with a band-aid or dry sterile dressing.

It is best not to burst a blister, because, till new skin grows, the skin over it helps to keep infection away.

WHEN TO SEE A DOCTOR

Seek medical help if the blister becomes red, hot, swollen, or filled with pus - this suggests an infection that may need treatment.

> Blister **ALERT!**
> - Pain
> - Fluid-filled lump under the skin
> - Clear fluid leaking from the blister

5 diarrhoea

Any type of irritation in the intestinal tract causes diarrhoea. The condition could be accompanied by abdominal pain and loss of appetite. Causes of diarrhoea can vary - food poisoning, drugs or medicines, or allergic reactions.

The most common danger from diarrhoea is dehydration. Your child loses a lot of fluid, vital body salts and minerals. If the condition persists, your child could become weak and exhausted. Sometimes, there may also be fever and sweating.

Treatment involves replacing lost fluids and minerals and attending to the cause of the problem.

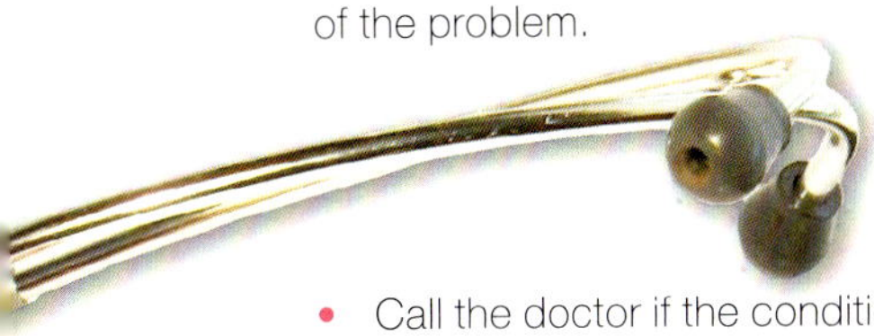

WHEN TO CALL A DOCTOR

- Call a doctor if the condition does not ease within 48 hours.
- Call the doctor if the condition appears to be an allergic reaction.
- Your child is not eating.
- There is fever or other symptoms accompanying the diarrhoea.

6 fainting

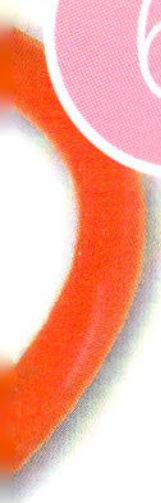

Fainting occurs because of a temporary reduction of blood flow to the brain. When the victim collapses, the natural blood flow to the brain is resumed, thereby helping to remedy the situation.

It is common for children to faint if they are very exhausted, or have been standing for long periods in the sun. Fainting may also be a reaction to emotional trauma or hunger.

WHAT YOU CAN DO

1. If your child is about to faint, get him or her to lie down. If the child is already falling, try to cushion the fall.
2. Raise your child's legs to improve blood supply to the brain.
3. Ensure a flow of fresh air.
4. Loosen tight clothing, especially around the neck and waist.
5. Reassure your child and help the child to sit up slowly.

Fainting **ALERT!**

- Signs of nausea with sweating
- Feeling light-headed
- Signs of giddiness

Always seek prompt medical attention.

7 nose bleeds

The blood vessels in the nasal lining are very fragile, so nosebleeds are a fairly common occurrence. These blood vessels can rupture with pressure, such as blowing the nose, or even sneezing.

Sometimes, being out in the hot sun for long periods can trigger a nosebleed. In children, this, and injury during sports are the common causes of nosebleeds.

WHAT YOU CAN DO

1. Ask your child to sit down, with the head tilting forward.
2. Tell your child not to talk and to breathe through the mouth.
3. Put a bowl under the nose and use a cloth to swab blood flow.
4. Gently pinch the nose, for about 10 minutes.
5. Release the pressure after 10 minutes. If the nose is still bleeding, press for another 10 minutes.
6. Once the bleeding stops, clean area with lukewarm water.
7. Make sure your child does not blow the nose.
8. If bleeding persists, call the doctor.

When in doubt, seek prompt medical attention.

8 sprains

Sudden, unexpected movements can lead to a tearing of muscles, known as muscle strain. When ligaments and tendons around joints are over-stretched, or tear, it causes a sprain.

Sprains create pain and tenderness around the joint. It is difficult to move the injured part of the body. There could also be localized swelling and bruising, indicating that the muscle or tendon may have ruptured. These soft-tissue injuries are sometimes hard to distinguish from fractures.

WHAT YOU CAN DO

Ask your child to relax, then follow the RICE procedure – Rest, Ice, Compression and Elevation.

- **R**est - do not allow your child to use the injured body part. Offer a soft pillow or other cushioned support.
- **I**ce - apply an ice pack or cold compress to reduce swelling in the area. If an ice pack is not available, try a pack of frozen peas, or similar packet, wrapped in a towel.
- **C**ompression – apply gentle pressure with soft, padded material, to reduce the swelling and bruising.
- **E**levation - If possible, raise and support the injured part, to reduce the blood flow in that area and minimize bruising.

When in doubt, seek prompt medical attention.

9 bumps & bruises

A bump or bruise is basically bleeding under the skin. Any blow to the body can cause this to happen, and the bruise may show up several hours after the impact. Most bruises heal by themselves.

Sometimes, a bump causes a swelling. On the scalp, because of the many blood vessels in this area, there is rapid swelling and you could see a large bulge. Most bumps and bruises are not serious but you should be alert for signs of more serious injury.

WHAT YOU CAN DO

1. Ask your child how the bump or bruise happened, as this can indicate the severity of the injury.
2. If it is a bump on the head, ask if your child lost consciousness at any time. If so, seek medical attention at once.
3. Raise the affected limb if possible and apply firm pressure.
4. Apply an ice pack for 5 to 10 minutes to reduce pain and swelling.

Always seek prompt medical attention.

10 home remedies

Very often, minor ailments have ready solutions in your kitchen "medicine chest". Spices, herbs, and other kitchen ingredients are very effective for some common problems. Listed here are typical problems that children have.

- indigestion
- diarrhoea
- nausea
- prickly heat
- over-strained eyes
- styes
- sore throat

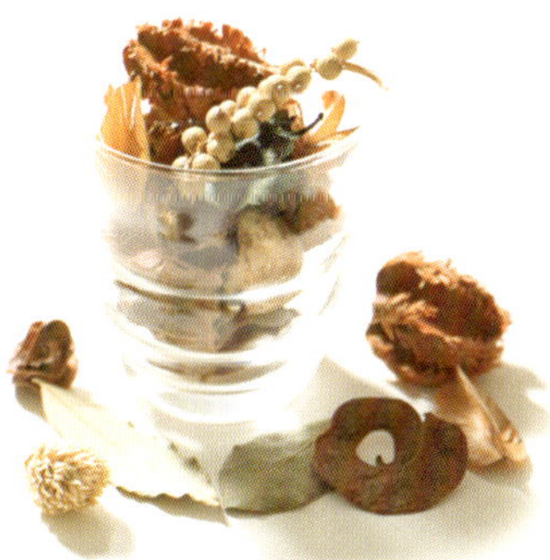

INDIGESTION

Over-eating and consuming unwholesome junk food can often lead to indigestion in children. Their small stomachs find it difficult to handle the excess food and a soothing home remedy can help to alleviate the symptoms.

Mix ginger and lemon juice, with a pinch of salt. Offer about 1 teaspoon at a time, at frequent intervals.

DIARRHOEA

A common problem in children. Watery stools cause dehydration and this is something to watch for. Children with diarrhoea need food and fluids, even if they appear to have diminished appetites.

- Rice khichadi or rice kanji is very effective. Rice kanji is made by cooking a handful of rice powder with water for 10 minutes, to make a thin liquid. Add a little salt and some more water, to desired consistency.
- A solution of salt, lemon juice, sugar and water can be frequently consumed.
- A glass of buttermilk, with a pinch of salt, helps fight germs and re-establishes the good bacteria.

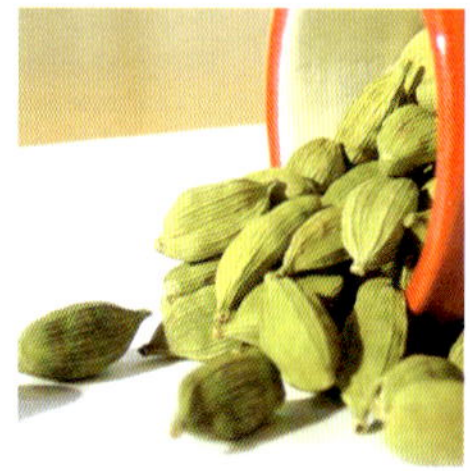

NAUSEA

Nausea itself is not a disease, but an unpleasant side effect of indigestion or an upset stomach. Consumption of contaminated food can lead to nausea, followed by vomiting. The symptoms can usually be treated with home remedies found in the kitchen.

- Ginger is a very effective anti-nausea treatment. Give your child juice of ginger, mixed with honey, to control the nausea.
- Offer green cardamom for chewing, to help control nausea.
- Dilute lime water with salt and sugar, offer it to alleviate nausea symptoms and ensure rehydration.
- Give older children peppermint tea.

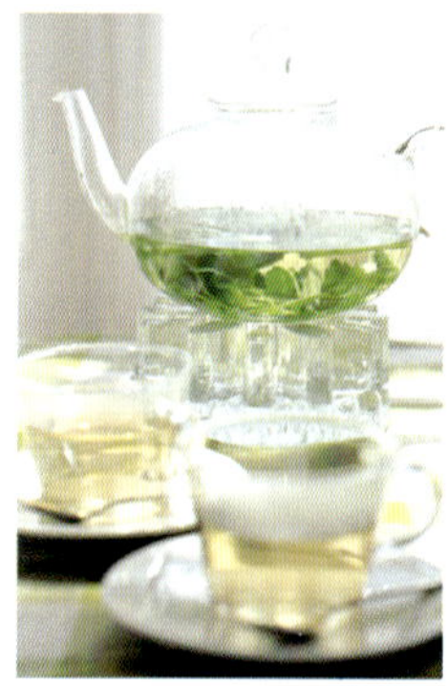

PRICKLY HEAT

Children have sensitive skins, vulnerable to heat and humidity. During the summer months, hot weather and internal body heat can cause prickly heat. The skin needs soothing, cooling remedies to alleviate the symptoms of rash and itchiness.

- Place aloe vera gel on the affected areas for a few minutes.
- Make a paste of sandalwood and rose water and apply on the rash area for instant relief.
- Make a paste of cornstarch and water and apply to the affected area. Once it dries, in about half an hour, it can be washed off with cold water.
- Give your child ample fluids, particularly cooling drinks like kokum sharbat and fresh lime juice to internally cool down the system.

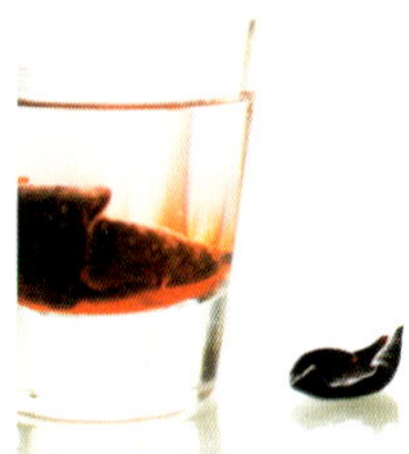

OVER-STRAINED EYES

In the age of television and computers, your child's eyes can often get red and strained. It is advisable to ask your child to take it easy for a while and keep the eyes shut. Some simple home remedies can ease eye strain in no time at all.

- Cut a cool cucumber into round slices and place over your child's closed eyes.
- Place used tea bags over the eyes for quick relief.
- Apply a poultice, with raw, grated apple in it. (A poultice is a little muslin cloth, filled with the required ingredient, and tied up.)
- Place cotton pads soaked in cold water over the eyes. This is an excellent way to refresh and relax the eyes and the surrounding tissues.

STYES

A stye could be a small painful boil, an inflamed hair follicle, or an infection of a sebaceous gland on the edge of the eyelid. When children have a stye, they tend to rub their eyes to relieve the itching, thereby spreading the infection from one hair shaft to another. This causes the stye to recurr.

Styes are infectious, so make sure you use a separate soap and face towel for your child.

- Use a warm water fomentation, 2-3 times a day, to relieve the affected eye.
- Mix ½ a teaspoon of boric powder with ¼ cup water. Use this solution to bathe the eye.

SORE THROAT

A sore throat can be a very persistent ailment, particularly in children. Anything from changes in the weather to too much shouting can trigger a sore throat. Treating it also requires persistence, and the remedies listed here, while not very tasty, are extremely effective.

- Add tulsi leaves to one cup water. Boil for 5 minutes. Strain and give your child this concoction to drink.
- Get your child to gargle with warm salt water.
- Offer hot milk with haldi mixed in it, to soothe the lining of the throat.
- Mix a spoon of honey with cinnamon powder and lime juice. Add a cup of hot water.

For information on dietary dos and don'ts relating to minor problems, log onto my website www.liveactive.com

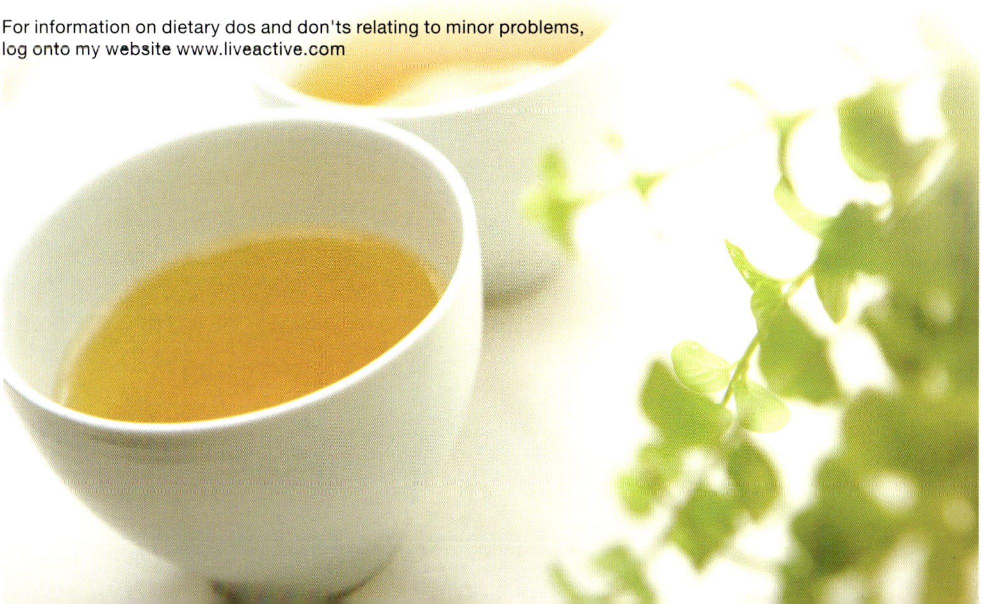